THURSDAY NIGHT THERAPY

Aaron M. Smith

THURSDAY NIGHT THERAPY

Thirty Years of Basketball and Camaraderie

AARON M. SMITH

TATE PUBLISHING
AND ENTERPRISES, LLC

Thursday Night Therapy

Published by Tate Publishing & Enterprises, LLC
127 E. Trade Center Terrace | Mustang, Oklahoma 73064 USA
1.888.361.9473 | www.tatepublishing.com

Tate Publishing is committed to excellence in the publishing industry. The company reflects the philosophy established by the founders, based on Psalm 68:11,
"The Lord gave the word and great was the company of those who published it."

Cover design by Jim Villaflores
Interior design by Caypeeline Casas

Published in the United States of America

ISBN: 978-1-63306-560-4
Sports & Recreation / Basketball
14.07.24

To all the men who have shown up under the lights for a little Thursday night therapy (and to the families that let them)

ACKNOWLEDGMENTS

Working on a book requires the support of so many, and I am thankful to the countless people who gave me their time, their expertise, and their encouragement during the process of transforming an interesting idea into this final product.

Many thanks go to my father-in-law, Fran Niehaus, and to the group of Thursday night hoopers, especially Wayne Jones, Jason Angelo, Roger Howell, Greg Van Dulman, John Orr, Mike Kraine, and Luke Howell. They not only welcomed me into their game but also provided me with stories and information from their experience in this thirty-year tradition. Special thanks also go to Pat Hanlon, Mike Brunner, and Fred Miller who took the time to tell me about their experiences with this group. Without these men, this game and this book do not exist.

I also want to thank Dr. Mark Smaller, Dr. Michael Zito, and Somatic Psychotherapist Brad Kammer for their time and expertise in providing me the psychological and psychoanalytical perspective of basketball. Their knowledge of their craft as well as their love of basketball added valuable insight to this story.

I have to thank my wife, Chrissy, for never blinking an eye when I leave on Thursday nights to go play basketball, sometimes with three kids still awake and showing no signs of tiring. I cannot adequately explain how much that means to me. I also would like to thank Chrissy for her unwavering support during the writing of this book. As I've said before, she is an incredible person to have in your corner.

Thanks go to my children, Sierra, Aidan, and Natalie. They provide the comedic relief that I need in my life and they come through on a daily basis. I would like to thank my parents, Scott and Monica, for their continued encouragement and inspiration. Thanks also go to my brothers, Jeremy and Nathanael, and my sister, Veronica, for their friendship and support. I would like to thank my mother-in-law, Peg Niehaus, for her encouragement and for watching my children so that I can have time during the week to write.

I want to thank Noel Thrasher, Rachael Sweeden, Wendee Lapating, Amefil Benguillo, and the many professionals at Tate Publishing for their interest, support, and expertise in transforming a computer document into this book. I always felt at ease working with this group of skilled and motivated individuals.

There are many others not mentioned above; it would take pages to mention everyone. If you helped me throughout the writing process, edited any of my work, allowed me into your establishments to write, showed interest in my work, played basketball with me, or encouraged me during the writing of this book, your kindness has not gone unnoticed. There is no way this book could have been written without so many generous and thoughtful people. Thank you all.

CONTENTS

PREFACE

> The invention of basketball was not an accident. It was developed to meet a need. Those boys simply would not play "Drop the Handkerchief."
>
> —Dr. James Naismith

James Naismith sat quietly in the office of Luther Gulick, glancing outside at the frosty New England morning. He scratched his mustache and gently shoved his glasses up the bridge of his nose and anxiously waited for Gulick to speak. Naismith knew this meeting had something to do with the increasing rowdiness of his students, but he was not quite sure about what to expect. Gulick sighed deeply, his fingers interlocked across his gray-vested belly.

"We've got to do something," Gulick finally said. The dapper gentleman, with a goatee the color of tree bark and a cloud-gray mustache, served as the director of physical education at the Springfield, Massachusetts, YMCA. Winter had gotten the best of his students, and he was running out of patience. "We need something to occupy this class of incorrigibles."

Naismith nodded in agreement. He was well aware that three previous instructors had failed to inspire these students; he hoped to himself that he would not be the fourth to be shown the door.

"I'd like you to come up with a winter game, one that can be played indoors," Gulick continued as Naismith listened intently. "These kids need an athletic distraction. They need a game that will keep them in shape for track, a game that is fair for all players, and a game that isn't so rough. You have two weeks to come up with something these children will play."

Naismith was no stranger to sport. Teaching and coaching a variety of sports to his YMCA students, Naismith was quite familiar with games such as football, lacrosse, baseball, soccer, and rugby. But those games were played outside. He needed something that could be performed on a smaller scale, one that could be played in the comforts of the gymnasium. He was confident he would be up to the challenge.

Naismith looked to his favorite games—football and soccer—as a starting point and tried to modify them for the indoor gymnasium. Certainly, these kids would enjoy this, he hoped. After failing miserably to create a proper modification of these games for the indoors, Naismith attempted to bring lacrosse into the gymnasium. Some of his students were from Canada and were experts at the game; however, the majority were decidedly not skilled enough and injured themselves. Naismith crumpled this idea like a mistake-filled rough draft and tossed it into a waste can across his office. He had to start from scratch.

Later that evening, the workings of Naismith's new sport began to formulate in his head. He wanted something similar to football but adamantly decided he would have no tackling, something that would be out of the question on the hard wood floors of school gymnasiums. He thought to himself, *But why is tackling necessary in football?*

He concluded that tackling was necessary because the players were allowed to run with the ball, and tackling was the means used to stop the runners. Naismith sat up at his desk and said aloud, "If he can't run with the ball, we don't have to tackle, and if we don't have to tackle, the roughness will be eliminated." He snapped his fingers and shouted, "I've got it!" It was Naismith's *eureka* moment.

One of Naismith's favorite games as a child was called Duck on a Rock, a game that combined tag and marksmanship. In this game, one player was required to stay near a stone—called the duck—in order to guard it from opponents. The other players would throw stones at the duck in an attempt to knock it off of a platform. Once it was knocked off, the throwers would rush to retrieve their stones. If a player was tagged before returning to the throwing line with his or her stone, they would become the guard. The guard could not tag anyone until he had picked up the duck at his feet, and he could not chase anyone until he had placed the original duck back up on its platform.

Naismith was fond of the idea of including marksmanship as a skill in his new game, but placing a guard in front of his goal would invite physical confrontations. This led the man to create one of his new rules that stated the goal would be placed above the players' heads in an attempt to reduce physical contact by making the goal *unguardable.*

With the basic premise of his new game in place—a ball [he had chosen a soccer ball because of its size and softness] and two goals placed high above the players' heads—Naismith began to fill in the blanks with how the game should be played and how it should be regulated by umpires and referees. Naismith located a pad of paper and began to scribble down what are now referred to as the original thirteen rules of Basket Ball.

1. The ball may be thrown in any direction with one or both hands.
2. The ball may be batted in any direction with one or both hands (never with the fist).
3. A player cannot run with the ball. The player must throw it from the spot on which he catches it, allowance to be made for a man who catches the ball when running at a good speed.
4. The ball must be held in or between the hands; the arms or body must not be used for holding it.
5. No shouldering, holding, pushing, tripping, or striking in any way the person of an opponent shall be allowed; the first infringement of this rule by any player shall count as a foul, the second shall disqualify him until the next goal is made, or, if there was evident intent to injure the person, for the whole of the game, no substitute allowed.
6. A foul is striking at the ball with the fist, violation of rules 3, 4, and such as described in rule 5.
7. If either side makes three consecutive fouls, it shall count a goal for the opponents (consecutive means without the opponents in the mean time making a foul).
8. A goal shall be made when the ball is thrown or batted from the grounds into the basket and stays there, providing those defending the goal do not touch or disturb the goal. If the ball rests on the edges, and the opponent moves the basket, it shall count as a goal.

9. When the ball goes out of bounds, it shall be thrown into the field of play by the person first touching it. In case of a dispute, the umpire shall throw it straight into the field. The thrower-in is allowed five seconds; if he holds it longer, it shall go to the opponent. If any side persists in delaying the game, the umpire shall call a foul on that side.
10. The umpire shall be judge of the men and shall note the fouls and notify the referee when three consecutive fouls have been made. He shall have power to disqualify men according to rule 5.
11. The referee shall be the judge of the ball and shall decide when the ball is in play, in bounds, to which side it belongs, and shall keep the time. He shall decide when a goal has been made and keep account of the goals with any other duties that are usually performed by a referee.
12. The time shall be two fifteen-minute halves, with five minutes rest between.
13. The side making the most baskets in that time shall be declared the winner. In case of a draw, the game may, by agreement of the captains, be continued until another goal is made.

When the allotted two weeks expired, Naismith walked into the cold gymnasium with his list of rules. Naismith took some clear tape from his office and fastened his rules to the gymnasium wall. He hurried over to the building superintendent and asked if the man had two boxes about eighteen inches square. The superintendent did not but offered Naismith two peach baskets from the storeroom that had no use. *Those would do just fine*, Naismith thought. He volunteered two students to take the peach baskets and secure them to the railings, which were about ten feet above the gymnasium floor, with a couple of nails. As the students studied the rules, trying to figure out what their teacher wanted them to do, Naismith divided his class into two teams of nine players. Naismith needed one more thing. He scurried out into the hallway and found a janitor quietly mopping the floors.

"Come with me," Naismith said, lightly grasping the man by his elbow. "I'm going to need you."

The game tipped off and Basket Ball was born. With every made shot, the janitor was summoned to the gallery to remove the soccer ball from the peach basket and toss it back down to the players. It would be some time before Naismith realized he could simply cut out the bottom of the baskets. After the game, Naismith reflected on his invention and scribbled down his initial thoughts about the first time Basket Ball was played.

> The class did not show much enthusiasm but followed my lead…I then explained what they had to do to make goals, tossed the ball up between the two center men & tried to keep them somewhat near the rules. Most of the fouls were called for running with the ball, though tackling the man with the ball was not uncommon.

The more these "incorrigibles" played this game, the more they enjoyed it. Word of the game made it to nearby schools and athletic clubs and visitors increasingly flocked to watch this new game. The sport was described by some as an "uproarious game accompanied by much yelling and undignified cheering." You could call it madness. Naismith, however, fell in love with his game and continued to modify his invention as his students improved at playing this sport, working out any inconveniences he found.

The year was 1891 and the world of sports—unbeknownst to Naismith—was about to change forever.

MORE THAN A GAME

How could Naismith have known? His chaotic game in the cold gyms of Massachusetts was nothing more than an "athletic distraction" from the long, bitter winters of New England. It was something to simply fill the void between the football and baseball and soccer seasons. But his sport exploded. That "class of incorrigibles" fell in love with the game also, and by 1892, the popularity of the sport had taken off on campus.

Dennis Horkenbach, the editor-in-chief of *The Triangle*, the Springfield College newspaper, featured Naismith's sport in an article called "A New Game." There were calls to name this new game "Naismith Ball," but the founder of the game refused the moniker. The game was officially called basketball instead and was introduced internationally by the YMCA movement in 1893.

More than 120 years later, basketball is a global enterprise. The sport is played every four years in the summer Olympics and has yielded some of the world's most recognizable athletic superstars.

But there is more to the game that Naismith drew up simply to fill a need for his rowdy students. There is more to it than international popularity and megastars and economic windfalls. The game is played in yards and lots all over the country, from the picturesque villages of Indiana and Ohio to the swarming streets and playgrounds of Los Angeles and New York.

Young boys and girls play the sport with peers or individually. Many tales have been told of the greats of the game shooting solitarily on their makeshift basketball goals in vacant barns or frigid driveways. Where there are no basketball rims, old milk crates are fastened to posts or tall trees and more than adequately serve their purpose. Friends gather to play after school or on weekends. Adults re-live their own childhood days by playing pick-up basketball games after work. The game has become therapy to some, an excuse for exercise and camaraderie.

In New Rochelle, New York, a group of men have been tying shoelaces and slipping into various forms of braces and wraps since 1971, all in preparation for their regular Saturday game in an old elementary gymnasium that looks like it could have been the setting for the movie *Hoosiers. ESPN.com* writer Eric Neel spent time with this group for an *ESPN.com E-Ticket* feature story about how powerful the bonds of basketball can be for those who relish community. And that's what a group of basketball players is really—a community.

Neel opined about how he once was part of a group of guys that played basketball regularly, even playing a game or two on the day of his wedding. But, sadly for Neel, he and his friends no longer get together to play basketball. His time spent with this group from New Rochelle showed Neel just what he had been missing. Basketball had become more than a sport to these men; it had become of way of life.

"We've all been enthralled by our experience in it," one of the regulars said in Neel's feature. "The game, how you play the game, the people you play with, that's who you are."

In 2010, *Washington Post* writer Lenny Bernstein wrote an article about a group of guys that had played every Sunday morning for twenty years in a local gym, complete with frigid temperatures and a slippery, dusty court. Bernstein quoted the leader of the group as saying, "The longevity comes from a perfect storm of love for the game, competitiveness, chemistry and a consistently solid run."

There is a difference between pick-up basketball and a long-running game. In a pick-up game, the rules are pretty standard. The game is to eleven, win by two. Make it, take it. Winners stay. Strangers come and go, teams are different, chemistry lacks. Showmanship trumps basketball. Talk outduels performance. But in a regular game against mostly familiar competition week in and week out, the games are a little different. Each game has its own rules set forth by the founder or by the group as a whole. The familiarity, though, is what makes the game special.

"There is a kind of civility," one of the players about whom Bernstein wrote, said. "You're playing with everyone day in, day out. You can't get too angry or belligerent. It wouldn't work."

And there is yet another game in New Jersey on an outdoor court in a public park. This game has been going on for twenty-nine years. The core has remained; others have come and gone, but the game has stayed the same. Sports Psychologist Dr. Michael Zito has played in this Friday evening game for all three decades. He plays with a group of friends and acquaintances, some of whom he has known since their basketball-playing days in kindergarten.

"It's really been something we look forward to and we arrange our lives around it to make it happen," Dr. Zito said. "It's a neat thing."

There are regular games all over the country. Some meet in the morning hours before work, others try to squeeze in a game at lunch, and others play in gyms or under the lights in the evening when the kids have gone to bed. Each game is unique—a blend of culture, religion, and life philosophy. For some, the regular game is simply guaranteed exercise. For others, it serves as an opportunity to get together with friends, or step away from their familial responsibilities, even if just for a few hours. And to others, it is a necessity, a slice of heaven on earth. To these men, missing a game for any reason is practically a sin.

A few miles north of downtown Cincinnati, there exists such a game. Vacations have been planned around Thursday nights. Work is put on hold until Fridays. Thursday night football games or must-see TV on the flat screen? Forget about it.

For thirty years, this game has continued, week in and week out. Many of the original players still arrive weekly, while a new crop of players has moved in to receive the baton, so to speak. This story is about that group, about that game, and about the psychological and emotional need for this game that inspires and motivates us to continue playing. For three hours every Thursday night, be it frigid or wet or humid or blazing hot, men of all ages and backgrounds convene under the lights of Apple Ridge Lane for a night that they will talk about or think about until the next Thursday night.

James Naismith may have simply created the game of basketball to keep some rowdy kids under control. But what he really did was create a way of life, a necessary recess from reality, for generations of incorrigibles to come.

INTRODUCTION

> Strive to build a team filled with camaraderie and respect: comrades in arms.
>
> —John Wooden

Fran Niehaus stands at just about five foot six, his ankles wrapped in braces, his feet nestled into extra wide black New Balance high-tops and multiple pairs of socks. He covers his bald head with an old triathlon hat that is missing half of the bill, which he cut off so that he could shoot a basketball without interference. Fran swears to himself that he'll be more than a foot taller sometime in another life.

"Dear, God, please make me six foot ten when I get to heaven," he'll say. "I'll even settle for six foot eight."

He's joking, sure, but I honestly think he has prayed to God to transform his frame into that of an NBA body when he reaches the great basketball court in the sky. I, for one, am a little afraid of this. I am six foot one and have had my share of blocks on Fran. After many of the swats, he will respond with an anguished snarl, "You dog!"

I am his son-in-law. And I am in trouble. If I am lucky enough to one day make it to heaven, Fran will make it hell on me on the holiest of courts.

Fran and I have a bond, certainly as in-laws, but likely even stronger as fellow basketball players. It is a bond my dad, Scott, formed with me at an early age, one that was nurtured under the hot summer sun on our gravel makeshift court an hour outside of Columbus, Ohio.

Some of my fondest memories are the grueling two-on-two games with my dad and my brothers, Jeremy and Nathanael. My love for basketball was born on that rock-infested court, which likely is the source of the ankle problems that plague me to this day. On that court, I was Ohio State's Jay Burson, Dennis Hopson, or Jimmy Jackson. I was Indiana Pacers guard Reggie Miller, shooting impossible three-pointers. I was anyone I wanted to be on that court. Growing up playing basketball with my dad and brothers and now playing with my father-in-law has given a special value to the game, transforming it into something much more than simply a sport.

I met Fran in 2004, and early on, my efforts were split between playing basketball and persuading him to allow me to date and eventually marry his oldest of three daughters, Chrissy. He relented on my persistence to marry his daughter, but he has yet to relent on the basketball court.

For nine months, I even lived with the man in transition before moving to California with Chrissy after our wedding in June of 2005. I left my job as a sports editor at the *Port Clinton News Herald* in October of 2004 and went to work for Fran until the following June, helping out with writing projects he needed for his law and financial planning office. I lived in his house for those nine months to save money for the upcoming cross-country move and, during that time, I played a lot of basketball with Fran. A lot of basketball.

We have endured exhausting one-on-one battles on the court together. What Fran may lack in height, he makes up for with quickness, endurance, and shooting accuracy. In the earlier days, he made me pay for being out of shape. I was about 212 pounds when I first started playing against Fran. I was a wheezing mess and struggled to stay with him. Those early games motivated me to get healthier, to shed that lazy bachelor weight that had been piling on since college. Now, thirty pounds lighter, I have closed the speed gap between us a bit and finally have the endurance needed to stay with Fran defensively.

We have frustrated each other, annoyed each other, and left each other shaking our heads. The game has squeezed out of us a few words that we would otherwise never say. That's basketball. That's competition. And we thrive on it.

It was about ten years ago also that I began playing with Fran and his longtime friends on Thursday nights. I'm one of the newer guys. Fran has been playing on Thursdays since 1984 on his very own court of dreams. I turned five years old then, and it was the year I received my first basketball for my birthday. Some of the guys Fran began playing basketball with thirty years ago still show up to battle under the Thursday night lights of Apple Ridge Lane.

After all, we all need a little therapy from time to time. We just don't need to lie on a couch to get it.

Thursday night basketball is a necessity for me. By the time it rolls around, the stresses of the week are just about at their peak. I am blessed; I am sensible enough to know that my stresses pale in comparison to some. That being said, being home with three children ages seven and younger a lot of the week while squeezing in time to write and take care of our house, my mind and body are in serious need of competition, male camaraderie, and an all-out physical challenge.

I've never been more exhausted than I am at about 12:05 early Friday morning after three hours of rigorous exercise on unforgiving concrete. Nothing, however, feels better than that fatigue, than that pain screaming in my ankles and knees, or wherever I received an errant elbow on that particular night.

I love the group of players we have on Thursday night. We have guys in their sixties who come complete with confounding energy and deadly accuracy. We have guys in their fifties and forties who shoot hook shots and try to implement spread offenses. We have guys in their thirties or younger who like to drive to the basket because they never were allowed to [or able to] when they played in high school. And, on occasion, a teenager [most likely a son or even grandson of one of the guys] shows up to play; his rabbit-like quickness and leaping ability an unfortunate reminder of just how old we're all getting.

It is a good mix of better people.

"I love being around people and I cherish community," Jason Angelo, a good shooter in his forties and one of our regulars for several years, said. "That's what's differentiated Fran's Thursday night hoops from anywhere else I've played. These are really, really good people. All walks of life, all age groups, all levels of skill, but totally consistent in the quality of character. And you couldn't pull together a nicer group of gentlemen."

The competition is great too. Everyone has their strengths. We have shooters and rebounders, lockdown defenders, and good passers. In a best-of-three series, we almost always go the distance.

Sure, there are times, though, when tempers can flare—a bad call here, a misplaced elbow there, a complaint or two that rises above a mutter.

But that is the nature of the sport. You can't battle against the same people for years and years under black muggy skies without getting into a bit of a disagreement from time to time. It's actually a blessing. We give each other an outlet, a way to release frustrations. The emotion comes out on the court instead of at home and that can only be a good thing.

"There'd be nights when you just want to hit somebody very hard or set a pick and nail somebody with a pick when they didn't see it coming," Fran admitted. "It was just to get some of that aggression out. It became like a fix to get that aggression out every Thursday night and it was a lot of fun."

I can relate. Sometimes, I can get worked up on the court. I get frustrated at myself and a week's worth of stress can pour out on the court. But that's good. I leave it on the court and feel like a burden has been lifted from my weary shoulders. No disrespect is ever intended, and I never feel disrespected when others release similarly. I believe there is an understanding, and we all need that "fix" as Fran called it.

The guys who show up on Thursdays are great men—businessmen, writers, lawyers, volunteers, and, more importantly, husbands and fathers. There may be a spat here or there, but I know that there is a great deal of respect for everyone that steps out there on that court. Nothing is ever personal. Nothing ever leaves the court.

"Like they say, I would be in the foxhole with any of them and I think, I hope, they would say the same about me," John Orr said, strong and stocky yet with a friendly face. He has been with this group from the start. "It's just been a pretty extraordinary run for thirty years and with a different cast of characters through the years. It seems that everyone who becomes involved with this group is just a super person."

To be expected, there have been injuries too. Broken fingers, torn ligaments, knees that bend in the wrong direction, broken noses, rolled ankles, teeth marks on balding heads, skinned knees, and separated shoulders. We are a tangle of wraps, braces, and sports goggles.

But we always come back.

Thursday night hoops is the equivalent of three hours of therapy every week. We all have problems ranging from health issues to work stress to family situations. It simmers and builds during the week and somehow, some way, there needs to be a release.

Thankfully, for all of us, Thursday night is always just around the corner.

TRADITION IS BORN

> Basketball is not just a metaphor for life—it is more important than that.
>
> —Engraving on a plaque in Phil Jackson's office

Slowly driving up and down streets in a small, tight-knit neighborhood north of downtown Cincinnati, Fran Niehaus peered into yards that had For Sale signs, and he envisioned a game of basketball being played between him and his friends. He could hear the ball bouncing on the ground, the sliding of high tops, the rub off of the wooden backboard, and—more importantly—the delightful swish of leather splashing through nylon.

"Too small," he said, passing one house with nowhere near enough space for a basketball court. "Wouldn't work with that one," he said, passing another.

He finally came across a home that was just right. It had an above-ground swimming pool that he knew his three daughters would love. There was a swing and room for badminton and volleyball. And, being on a double lot, it had more than enough room to contain Fran's basketball court.

One problem—there was no For Sale sign. No realtor to call. No reasonable clue as to who lived there or if anyone inside would be interested in selling the place.

Issues like that, though, didn't really bother Fran. He saw those situations as challenges, as opportunities.

Winton Place was a small area—two or three blocks by ten blocks—and the attraction to the neighborhood for Fran and his wife Peg was the New Jerusalem Community, which was founded by Richard Rohr, OFM. Rohr was a Franciscan friar and internationally known speaker and author and served as the pastor of this community. He had made Winton Place the center of the group, which was comprised of roughly two hundred people, most of whom were in their late twenties to early thirties. People in New Jerusalem had flocked to Winton Place during the previous five years and houses there were in great demand. Community members had purchased what they could and many people were still looking for homes in the area. Fran and Peg were determined to move to Winton Place; they knew where every community member lived on every street in the neighborhood. Their criteria for a home were two-fold: Was there a community member living in the house and, if not, was there enough room for a basketball hoop?

The house with the pool and a double lot was just one of twenty houses they wrote on a list of potential homes. Once their drive through the neighborhood was complete, Fran penned a letter to send out to each of the owners:

> Dear Owner,
>
> My wife and I and three children are interested in moving to Winton Place. We drove by your house, and it seemed like it would meet our needs. If you are interested in selling, I'd appreciate your contacting us. Thank you.
>
> Sincerely,
> Fran Niehaus

Time passed and trips to the mailbox were fruitless. One afternoon, as Fran flipped through the envelopes in his mailbox, he noticed a letter with the return address: 716 Derby. The house with the pool. The house with plenty of room for Fran's hoop dreams. The only house on their list with the word *nice!* scribbled beside the address.

For more than twelve years, Fran had been living in a home devoid a basketball court while Peg had watched as her family's second-floor dwelling in a two-family brick house shrank around her. Both had the same need to move, but Fran wasn't prepared to okay any potential new house that didn't have the space he needed.

"I only had one requirement," he said with a smile. "It had to have room for a basketball court."

They opened the envelope and pulled out the letter. With great delight, Fran and Peg read that the owners were interested in selling the property. And when the dust settled and paperwork was all signed, Peg finally got her one-family house with ample space, and Fran got his basketball court.

The year was 1984, and Thursday night hoops was about to tip-off.

THURSDAY NIGHT HOOPS

Before Fran ever anticipated his first game at the house, the seed of Thursday night hoops had already been planted and cultivated on a backyard court in North Bend, Ohio. Pat Hanlon, a big, bruising former college football player who could play a little basketball too, was a player in a regular basketball game on Thursday nights in the late 1970s. He was strong and forceful in the lane, a dominating presence.

He considered himself a basketball player even though many still remember him only as a football player who could play a little hoops too.

"Sports were in my blood," Pat said. "Everywhere I ever lived, I had to have a basketball hoop."

In 1979, a divorce sent Pat from North Bend to Winton Place, the small neighborhood tucked in the valley near Spring Grove just off of Interstate 75 a few miles north of downtown Cincinnati. Basketball was one of the most effective distractions that helped keep Pat's mind off of the divorce.

"The first thing I did at that place was build a basketball court," Pat said. "It wasn't the best, but I needed to play. I picked up playing on Thursdays because that's when I played in North Bend. I started playing with guys in the neighborhood, and it became pretty regular."

A few years passed and Pat married a woman from the community and moved "about five houses down the street." There was one problem, however.

"I tried to put up a hoop there, but there just wasn't enough room," he remembered. "We had to start playing down at the schoolyard whenever we could."

This went on until 1984 when Fran's need for a basketball court revived Thursday night hoops on a double lot off of Derby with a swimming pool as instant relief after games played in sweltering Cincinnati evenings. Thursday became the official night of basketball because the New Jerusalem Community members had their small group meetings on Mondays or Tuesdays and on Wednesdays, they gathered for worship.

"Thursday night was the logical night to play for us," Fran said. "I did not really know about Pat having played on Thursday nights regularly before."

The Niehauses moved into their new home on October 1, 1984 and, as movers lumbered in and out of the house with furniture on their backs, Fran walked the driveway, configuring the court in his head. Once it was settled where all was to go, Fran hired a company to help him weld a pole and backboard support that would allow his basketball hoop to stand the test of time. He had two requirements for his setup. The first was that the backboard had to be regulation size.

"I didn't want any part of one of those half-moon-shaped backboards because I liked to use the entire backboard," Fran said. "The moon shape always wreaked havoc with my bank shots."

There was already a small goal on the lot—a six-foot hoop that leaned. Fran said it was good for dunking, but that it had a half-moon backboard. There was no way he was going to recycle that backboard for his court. He was going to construct his own backboard out of marine wood and it would be at regulation size. The new basket was placed so that the slight slope angled toward the would-be free throw line. "This was so the balls would naturally bounce back to you," Fran explained.

Fran's second requirement was that the hoop needed to be able to withstand wind and weather and anything else for years to come. A pole was engineered for the hoop that was secured more than five feet in the ground in a foundation of cement. More than fifteen bags of cement were used in the gaping crater to secure the pole. One of the neighbors and a regular basketball player who helped with the project was convinced a nuclear bomb would not be able to topple the structure.

The project was a multiday affair, and Fran doggedly patrolled the court with a measuring tape, a level, and a vision until everything was the way it had appeared to him that day while driving slowly through the neighborhood. Tiny metal washers were placed behind the rim, one by one, until the rim was exactly level from every spot on the court. If it was just a millimeter off, Fran would not have been able to sleep at night.

"Fran is a bit anal when it comes to the hoop," Wayne Jones, a great athlete and one of the original players that still comes out every week, joked. "The backboard and rim are ready. The pole has been set in cement. Fran has his tape measure. Everyone helps to get the goal in the exact location. It must be the exact distance from the ground, from the end line, and must be perfectly set before we're done."

Then the players had to pour the concrete in the court area that wasn't already covered in asphalt. The work had been laborious enough without young children running around, but Fran's oldest daughter, Chrissy, escaped into the working area. Just six years old at the time the concrete portion of the court was poured, she couldn't contain her excited energy—something that hasn't changed today—and ran through the wet cement. Greg Van Dulman saw the entire thing unfold as if it were in slow motion; however, his pleas for Chrissy to stop were too late.

"I just remember him, yelling, 'Get off of the court!' at the top of his lungs," Chrissy said. "'What are you thinking!' They had to do it all over again. They were all pretty mad at me, but I remember Greg really getting upset."

"I don't think I got *that* upset," Greg recalled with a smile. "I just remember seeing her coming, and I was on the other side of the court. I had to say something and a 'honey, don't' wasn't going to work in that situation.

"I will say that I did apologize to her afterward," Greg said with a laugh.

Once the footprints were smoothed over and the concrete had cured, the games could finally begin. Initially, the court did not have a three-point line and all rebounds had to be taken back out to the top of the key. At the time, three-point lines were only used in the NBA. They hadn't been added to college or high school courts and wouldn't be added until 1986 [NCAA] and 1987 [high school], respectively.

Because of Thanksgiving and Holy Thursday, the guys played their game on Wednesdays those two weeks. Once three-pointers became commonplace in basketball, Fran would chalk a temporary three-point line on the court on Wednesdays, but "because I love shooting threes, it felt a little like a self-serving situation to have threes on Thursday nights and count by twos and threes [instead of by ones]."

But after a few of those Wednesday nights, the players agreed to have a permanent three-point line painted on the court for their Thursday night game. The players loved the opportunity to shoot threes; it was an option that opened up the court because the ball could then be taken out on all sides. It created more scoring opportunities and allowed for a better chance at coming back on a team. Just as the three-point line revolutionized the college and pro games, it transformed the way the Thursday night game was played.

Garage lights and a single flood light attached to a nearby tree provided the illumination for the court so that the game could go deep into Thursday night and into the early morning hours of Friday. It was perfect. Expect for maybe the height of the light.

"The garage light wasn't quite high enough," Fran remembered. "There was a blind spot when passes came from the corner. That created some panicked reactions when someone would do a bullet pass."

The game continued on at Derby, one Thursday night at a time through wind, through rain, through heat, and through frost for nearly a decade. But as Fran's family continued to grow up, the need for a new house once again became a priority. And for Fran, there was no question about his needs with any new home. The search began but netted no reasonable results. They couldn't find a home with a quality basketball court.

One Saturday morning in 1993, as they lay awake in bed, Peg and Fran were brainstorming about possible places to move.

"You know, you can build your own basketball court," Peg said. "I went down to that new street and you couldn't hear the highway. I stood where the driveway would go, and I couldn't hear the cars. You could build your court there."

Fran quietly pondered what his wife had just told him. That new street was Apple Ridge Lane in Amberley Village, a quiet neighborhood about ten miles north of the city. The street was dotted with brand new upper-scale houses, and a home there would certainly meet the needs of his wife and his three daughters.

Fran's only question at that moment pertained to the property lines.

With the three-point line being nineteen foot nine inches from the center and needing two and a half to three feet for turnaround three pointers in the corner, I figure we'll need about forty-four feet, he thought.

Thirty minutes later, Fran and Peg were standing directly on the future site of Thursday night hoops. Upon review of the property lines and a careful calculation of the space needed for his court, Fran found that he would have just enough space, almost down to the inch. It must have been fate.

The game became such a commonality when it moved to Apple Ridge Lane, that Fran's neighbors came to use it as a reminder to put the trash out—Friday is trash day. However, those two Wednesday games sometimes threw the whole street off its routine.

"People got so used to Thursday night hoops that when we played on Wednesday nights, people would put their garbage out because they saw the lights on and people playing ball," Fran said. "They weren't thinking, and like Pavlov's dogs, they put their garbage out when they saw the lights. I did, too, on more than one occasion."

For thirty years now, the game has become a staple in our lives. When you wake up on Thursday mornings and go through the day's schedule in your head, a smile hits your face when you realize that it is basketball night. All of a sudden, there is an excitement and the adrenaline starts to course through your veins.

Basketball is a beautiful sport, especially when played correctly. And the game can only be played the right way by good people who understand it and all of its complexities. And it is those good people, the ones who consistently show up under any circumstance, the ones you can count on, who make this game the special tradition it has become to each of us.

THE PLAYERS: THE HEART AND SOUL OF THE GAME

> What you are as a person is far more important than what you are as a basketball player.
>
> —John Wooden

Jason's team had quickly tallied seventeen points on a flurry of outside shots and just needed a three-pointer to win the game. Breathing heavily yet still with a spring in his step, the program manager at Dunnhumby USA, stood ready at the top of the key, waiting for the ball to be checked. Jason, athletic and in his forties, had quality options: Fran was on his team and was one the group's best shooters. Wayne, too, was on Jason's team and had a penchant for hitting game-winning shots. And Jason had John. John was the key because his brick-wall of a body could keep possessions alive with rebounding, and when he was having a good night, he could consistently hit shots with the best of them. On that night, he had been on fire.

All four players had a realistic chance to end the game with a single shot, which isn't rare. We are all shooters on Thursday nights.

Roger had just given his team a one-point lead with an inside bucket, and his team was just a defensive stop and a two-point shot away from winning. I was on his team and had the responsibility of guarding Fran—a son-in-law versus father-in-law dynamic in full vigor. Neither one of us liked to lose to the other. Byron Heizer, strong and sturdy, needed to use his strength to keep John at bay, while Luke, Roger's twenty-four-year-old jumping-jack of a son, was covering Jason.

There are times when the team with seventeen points thinks they can still win by going in twos. That game was not the time to try that because Roger's team was scoring at will in the paint. Jason's group knew they needed a three-pointer to win, and they needed it right then because they did not want to let the other team have a chance.

"I think the odds of winning when you go for two in that situation are dramatically decreased," Fran said. "Once you go inside, they're not going to give you anything."

I'd have to agree.

Jason received the check from Luke, and the battle began. Picks came from both sides, and Jason drove to his left. The defense called for switches and desperately chased down any man close to them. Jason found Wayne who was quickly smothered. Picks and rolls and players cutting and dashing resembled the chaotic three-man weave drill during high school basketball practice. Someone was bound to come open. Our defense was stout, though. We were quick; no one came close to a clean look.

But sometimes, the best way to beat that defense is to take a chance. And that is what Jason did when he got the ball back on the right wing. He was covered well but heaved a long three-pointer over the outstretched hands of Luke who had come flying into the play after fighting through a pick. The ball bounced high off the back of the rim and then came down, scraping the front of the rim. There was a mad dash for the rebound; the team that came up with the ball would likely come out on top. The ball bounced off of a few fingers, but John secured the loose ball.

We were in trouble. Our defense had been compromised and someone was open. That someone was Fran. John sensed he had an outlet and fired the ball toward Fran. Roger and I scrambled and sprinted out toward the line. We were too late. Fran had enough time to release the shot over our outstretched hands. I didn't even look. I heard the flick of the net and the loud "Yeah!" from the winning squad and the high-fives that followed.

Game over. Twenty to eighteen.

My gut churned, and I tried not to look at the guys on the other team celebrating. I quickly walked to the top of the key and couldn't wait to start the next game; I needed to feel something else other than the frustration that was beginning to cloud my mind. I just stood there, waiting while others were getting drinks, a replay of every one of my missed shots and every pass I threw to the other team flashed in my mind. I felt that I had let my team down, and the pressure I had put on myself to be successful became an irritating burden.

Roger took the loss in stride, walking over to get a drink while shaking his head. He congratulated the other team and realized the great experience in which he just took part. Byron simply shook his head and smiled, understanding how great a game was just played. Luke, like his dad, headed over for water, but the disappointment was more apparent on his face than on Roger's.

During the years, I've noticed two types of reactions to the endings of games. I thought it simply boiled down to two types of people—those who like to win versus those who hate to lose. But it is more than that. It is a specific mindset of each individual that triggers his emotions and actions on the court in a given situation.

Personalities of the guys who play basketball in our group tend to emerge on the court. You can often tell how they are off the court by the way they play and how they react to the game. You can tell the guys who are more laid back and those who have tipping points. We have guys who are team players—the motion offense guys, and we have guys who are great finishers—the guys who crave that final shot. There are guys who hate to lose and it shows on their faces and in their determination to quickly start the next game. And there are guys who brush off a loss on the court as nothing more than an opportunity to improve.

FIXED VERSUS GROWTH MINDSETS

Dr. Michael Zito is a psychologist in New Jersey, and during the last fourteen years of his twenty-nine-year career, has studied and worked in the field of sports psychology. For three decades, he, too, has been a regular player in a long-standing game of basketball at a public park. He understands basketball as well as the mental side of the sometimes confounding game. In explaining the difference between guys who beat themselves up over a loss and the guys who let a bad game roll off of their backs like water off of a duck, Dr. Zito pointed to two particular mindsets: fixed mindsets and growth mindsets.

"Fixed mindset individuals define themselves in the here and now," Dr. Zito said. "So we won, we feel good. We lost, we feel bad. Compared to the growth mindset, which is more like [my mindset], I just want to improve my game. I don't feel a lack of success. I just want to work on the basics. Get my feet set, get square to the basket, participating, getting people involved. That's been me my whole life; I couldn't care less about losing. I'm more into enjoying the process."

The guys with the fixed mindset, according to Dr. Zito, have a tendency to define themselves by how they're playing or by the outcome of the game. He has seen players who have had a bad game or who lose a game and the anger or intensity of the loss can be seen and heard and felt by those around them. People with this particular mindset have a hard time not making the defeat personal. Criticism or bad play can be misinterpreted as criticism or a reflection of you personally.

I admittedly have demonstrated that fixed mindset on the basketball court, especially when I was younger. According to Carol Dweck, a psychologist and author who teaches at Stanford University, the difference between the fixed and growth mindset "isn't ability; it's whether you look at ability as something inherent that needs to be demonstrated or as something that can be developed."

People with the fixed mindset worry about their traits and how adequate they are. They have something to prove to themselves and others, Dweck wrote. I often feel like I have to prove myself in order to fit in to particular groups. When I have a good night on the court, I feel like I can be accepted. When I don't, however, I feel like my ability or my acceptance in the group has taken a hit or is being judged as inadequate. Especially on nights when a new player is coming, I feel like I have to establish myself as a good player in fear of being judged as inadequate if I have a bad night. I am later able to realize that that idea is ridiculous, but in the moment, I am constantly trying to prove myself.

I do not like to lose. Who does? But I have noticed that I hate losing more than I enjoy the feeling of victory. For me, the feeling associated with winning is only that of relief at not losing. In my mind, losing demonstrates a lack of ability or a lack of success. And when I am on a team that loses, I feel responsible. I tend to feel the heat lamp square on my face like a suspect being interrogated in a dimly lit cell. I often believe others are judging my abilities, both on the court and off of it.

I believe this self-imposed pressure to succeed stems from the struggles I endured trying to fit in with my high school basketball team nearly twenty years ago. I was generally thought of more as a science nerd [I once cloned alfalfa for a science fair project!] than a basketball player, and I certainly wasn't regarded as one of the more popular kids on the team—my enormous Chris Sabo Rec Specs and my timid personality at the time made me a bit of a target to some people the first couple years of high school. I was even bullied by some of my teammates during summer basketball camps and during the hours after school waiting for practice to begin. This demeaning treatment ignited in me an obsession with being accepted by those I deemed important. And, to me at the time, playing basketball at a high level meant being accepted. I wrongly felt that if I were to somehow score twenty points in a game, those who mistreated me would all of a sudden respect me. I like to think that I've matured a bit since then, but every now and then, those old feelings come back and feel as raw as a recently opened scab.

I tell myself before every night not to get too competitive at the end of games. I tell myself that it really isn't that big a deal losing these games—we're just here to have fun, release, and get a good workout in. Twenty minutes into the night, I've failed in my goal of not caring whether we win or lose. I'm back in high school again, trying to fit in, trying to feel included.

I can feel the sting of defeat in the pit of my stomach, especially when I've missed makeable shots or when we have more turnovers than shot attempts. It's just a backyard game, yet losing always seems to feel like something meaningful that was within grasp has just been ripped away. Yes, I realize that's absurd. However, a gain in perspective over the years—having children, natural maturation, etc.—has allowed me to see the bigger picture, more like those with a growth mindset.

Most of the guys we play with on Thursdays have this growth mindset. They see the big picture, much like Dr. Zito. They see the game for what it is. Those with a growth mindset understand that self-image is not tied to how well they shoot or whether or not they have had a few turnovers. Self-image is not married to how others view your performance. Failure is an opportunity to learn, not an indictment on you personally. This is where I have struggled.

"I don't care whether we win or lose, I'm getting exercise," Dr. Zito said. "That's really my focus. I don't define myself by, 'Did we win three games or not?' The goal is to get out there for some camaraderie and exercise. That's it."

The irony, I've discovered, is the less you try to impress people with the way you play basketball, the less you care about how others view your performance, the better you play. I wish I had understood this concept back in high school.

There is a notion out there that who you are on the basketball court is a reflection of who you are as a person. Craig Robinson, a former two-time Ivy League Player of the Year at Princeton and once a fourth-round draft pick of the Philadelphia 76ers, once played in a regular game with some friends and the competition was, obviously, pretty stiff. Craig's sister was dating a man and she wanted to see if he was the real deal. She knew basketball was a good way to view the inner workings of a person, to understand the truth about a person. She asked her brother if this man could play in Craig's game in order to get an idea about what type of guy he was. Craig agreed.

In his interview with Chuck Klosterman of *Esquire Magazine*, Craig described this man as "quietly confident, which means he had good self-esteem without being cocky. He was certainly a team player—he wasn't a pig, he passed when he was supposed to pass, and he cut when he was supposed to cut. To me, that speaks to a lack of selfishness. He had natural leadership ability, because he didn't just pass me the ball because he was dating my sister. Whenever a player gets tired, he reverts back to the player he truly is. That's how you tell. And we played for hours. That's how I could tell."

That player was future President of the United States, Barack Obama.

In addition to mindset differentiation, Dr. Zito explained that there are two broad types of people as it relates to personalities being carried over into sports: "Those who are consistently the same and those that are able to flex given the needs of the situation." In other words, there are some players whose personalities off the court mirror their play on the court.

There are also those who may show a higher level of intensity in the sports arena when the situation demands it.

"Some people are consistently one way and others can be flexible and turn it on in some situations," Dr. Zito explained. "For example, Derek Jeter, is a pretty calm exterior kind of guy, but when he needs to, he turns it on and does what he needs to do to get the job done.

"One of the guys we play with, I've known since age five," Dr. Zito continued. "He's kind of an intense kind of guy. He's pretty much always intense. He bangs heads with people on the court; he'll dive for loose balls. He doesn't always fluctuate. For me, I'm kind of always relaxed, I'll be reasonably aggressive on the court, you know, within the limits of a fifty-four-year old body. But I'm not wanting to go diving into something though."

Basketball can be a good indicator of who you are off the court; it often can reveal a player's strengths and weaknesses. Our Thursday night group in Cincinnati is no different. We are a group of varied characters with different backgrounds and philosophies on life. Those characteristics and traits show up in ways that are very recognizable to anyone who has played a regular game of basketball or even in a recreation league at a local gym.

CAST OF CHARACTERS

Scott Gordon could have been a coach. He understands the intricacies of spatial movement on the basketball court unlike anyone since Norman Dale coached the Hickory

Huskers to a fictional Indiana state championship in the movie *Hoosiers*.

"We need motion!" Scott often shouted, crouching with the ball in his textbook triple-threat position at the top of the key. "We need cutters!"

I can see Dale's philosophy take shape every time Scott has the ball. Scott, looking younger than his age would indicate, loves to see four passes before any shots are taken—before anyone even thinks about taking a shot. When he shows up on a Thursday night, you just know how his team will play.

"Five players on the floor functioning as one single unit," Dale preached to his undermanned high school squad in the movie, *Hoosiers*. "Team, team, team—no one more important than the other." I would like to point out that, as team-oriented as it sounds, Dale's philosophy didn't really work until Jimmy Chitwood and his incredible shooting touch joined the team halfway through the season. In all those game montages in the movie, you rarely saw Jimmy pass the ball.

Scott, who no longer plays regularly with our group, sometimes ran Dale's philosophy to a fault. You see, Scott was one of the best shooters in our group and one of our best athletes. He had broad shoulders and was sturdily built with hardly a pound of body fat. His arms alone could effectively box out a defender. To top it off, his shooting touch was pure. When he would get on a roll, there was nothing a defender could do about it. But there were times when he would come off a pick and receive the ball about twelve feet from the basket. Unguarded, he would stand there and call for cutters so that he could find someone for a closer shot. He was Princeton in the UCLA world of backyard basketball.

"I'll never understand it," Fran said. "Take the shot! You're wide open!"

Fran isn't very vocal on the court, usually only audibly chastising himself over a poor shot attempt. I think the only times we've heard him yell at another player is when Scott passed up an open look.

Scott was one of, well, probably the only one in our group that we would all harp on to shoot more.

In 2007, Patrick Hruby, a writer at *ESPN.com,* wrote a comical article that accurately depicted some of the stereotypical guys you see in pick-up basketball games. As I was reading this, I started to see just how some of our players fit into the basketball family.

I've already mentioned one of the characters—"The Coach on the Floor." Scott most definitely fit into this category. We could win a game 20–13 and Scott would end the game shaking his head because we didn't have good spacing or someone didn't rotate. We used to kid him about it, sure, but we rarely admitted that the game did have better flow when he was there.

Another category that Hruby wrote about was "The Guy Who Doesn't Know His Own Strength." We have a couple of guys that fit this mold, but probably no one more so than "Big" Mike Kraine. He is roughly six feet tall, but his arms are as thick as my legs. His dusty brown wavy hair sits atop his chiseled face. He is gritty and powerful, likely a better linebacker than a shooting guard.

Mike was as graceful as Dick Butkis on ice skates. When he played regularly, Mike had two moves—a "wicked" spin move into a fade away, as he called it, or the power drive to the right side of the lane. As a defender, you prayed for the spin move. Only one person has ever attempted to take a charge from Big Mike, and he left the game with a broken wrist never to return.

"He can control the boards because he can control anyone around him with those iron-like arms," Fran said. "He got better and better at shooting as time grew on, even developing that little lefty off of the turn-around dribble."

Mike was a guy who would think he was simply boxing you out, playing his role as a rebounder. But if you were the one he was boxing out, you thought Mike had a problem with you for some reason. You wondered why you were six feet out of bounds sliding in mulch that Fran's wife had just put down in the garden. You wondered why your reversible jersey had been reduced to nothing more than a rag to wash your car. Mike knew he was strong; I just don't think he realized how much stronger than the rest of us he actually was when he played.

Before there was Mike, Pat Hanlon was the guy who didn't know his own strength. John Orr, one who certainly uses his strength as an asset, said Pat was tough to guard because you couldn't anticipate what he was going to do on the court.

"He was a bit of a bull in a China shop kind of player," John recalled. "He had a bit of a colorful personality too. He reminded me of my brother, who was more football oriented. As I'm reflecting, I kind of feel like I'm turning into Pat these days.

"Although [the other players] assured me it's not to that point yet," he added with a chuckle.

Then there is the "Marathon Man." This guy does not come equipped with an "off" switch. Hruby wrote: "If the

Marathon Man doesn't compete in actual marathons—or triathlons, bicycle road races, swimming the English Channel or some other ungodly test of human endurance—then he's currently training to do so. Which means he's in shape. Tremendous shape. Better shape than you, better shape than everyone else on the court."

Fran is our Marathon Man. This wiry yet sturdy man in his sixties is not intimidated by Father Time. At 11:58 in the evening, when many of us are dry heaving or lying flat on our backs in the middle of the court waving at floating white spots that only we can see, Fran can be heard gleefully asking, "Who's staying?"

"At sixty-three years old, he's in better shape than most of the guys who play," Wayne said. "And he'll probably still be playing at eighty."

That's not hyperbole. He would rather go for a five-mile hike than watch a game on television. A television show that made history? Fran has no time for that. There's an empty basketball court somewhere just begging for a game to be played.

"*Seinfeld* was quite a show," Fran said, though he admitted he never really watched the Thursday night can't-miss and award-winning show. "While *Seinfeld* was on TV doing its thing to the world, I was out playing Thursday night hoops."

Fran trains for the Little Miami Triathlon, which he often runs twice a year (six miles of canoeing, six miles of running, and eighteen miles of biking, anyone?). He said he runs the triathlons to stay in shape for basketball. It's working.

We've also got "The Braveheart," the guy who "never calls a foul, even when there is blood and/or human entrails on the court," Hruby wrote.

Our Braveheart would be Roger Howell. Roger is our true post player, although he's recently developed a long-range shot, much to our dismay. He is thin and plays much taller than his actual height of just over six feet; his lengthy reach causes grief all over the court. He is a proud card-carrying member of the old school—the Kevin McHale brand of old school. When the ball goes into the post, it doesn't come back out, no matter what grisly triple-team awaits him in the lane.

Roger is constantly getting beat up out on the court, yet he continues to pound away on the inside. He'll often turn with the ball and go up for a closely contested shot. He will get drilled in the waist by a shorter guy. His arm will be smacked by another—the sound of which echoes down the street. The off-the-ball defender will usually come flying in for the block and send Roger's sleek sports glasses hurtling toward the concrete as the shot soars just left of the mark.

"Oh, Roger!" He'll yell at himself for not making the shot.

No foul called. Nothing. We usually just stop playing, expecting him to call a foul, but all we often hear is Roger lamenting his own miss and the echo of coyotes yelping in the distant green space. He is as tough as they come, often playing with wrapped knees, taped fingers, and bandaged ribs. He earns every point he gets out there on that court.

We've had to start calling our own fouls against Roger because there is no way he'll call them. Respectable, of course. Unless if he's on your team. In that case, call the bloody foul!

We also have many a Glad-Hander in our group, the masters of the growth mindset. This player is generally all smiles. He complements everyone with "Nice shot...you're just an inch off...keep shooting...you'll get it." He's the guy who always defers judgment calls to the opposing team. He's self-deprecating. When he makes a shot, he's lucky. When someone else hits a shot, they're "on fire!" Hruby wrote, "After losses, Glad-Handers claim they're only in it for the exercise, an assertion that's a lot maddening and a little enviable."

Wayne Jones would be our lead Glad-Hander, and I mean this with about as much respect as I can offer. Wayne is probably my favorite person to play with on Thursday nights. His love for the game rubs off on all of us. It is that love affair with the game that keeps his perspective in check too.

"[When I was a kid] I spent hours playing by myself on the playground, announcing the game as I played against myself," he said. "If I wanted to work on my shot, I'd go to the monkey bars. I'd dunk between the bars or even work on shooting between them to hone my accuracy. At home I'd make a paper basket, tape it to the wall, and use a wadded sheet of paper to play in my room. I couldn't get enough of it during basketball season."

He appreciates every minute he has to play. Wayne is probably the nicest guy on the floor. He competes hard too; he's probably the best rebounder on the court. But after a loss—even a close, nail-biting, bitter, defeat—he'll tell the other guys how well they shot. He doesn't show a hint of despair at the loss.

"I'm a team player," Wayne said. He refers to our Thursday night game as his *happy place*. You would never guess Wayne is in his sixties; his dark hair and youthful face mislead you. "I may have my shining moments, but I'm more of a support player."

Then there are some stereotypes that Hruby did not write about. For instance, the Game Seven Guy. The fixed mindset guy. Me. I will say, however, that I am getting better at this. Maturity has a way of doing that. I'm not sure, though, that a loss will ever feel good. There have only been a few losses that brought a smile to my face.

One, for example, was when Big John had the ball a good twenty-seven feet from the basket. His team needed a three-pointer to win; I was on the team that was mounting an impressive comeback, so close to a great win. I was also guarding John. I was about as close to John as I could be without a foul being called. I didn't care that he was twenty-seven feet away from the basket. If a team needed a three-pointer, I was not going to let my guy get a clean look. John did not have a clean look. He took the shot regardless, much to my surprise. I jumped as high as I could. There really was no way John could see the basket. The shot soared high in the air. It began coming down, and I saw that it was somewhat on line. It couldn't. It did. The ball banked off of the dew-moistened backboard and went purely through the net. Game over. I just turned and looked at John in amazement as he simply strolled off of the court with a sheepish grin splashed on his face. I couldn't help but smile. Sometimes, there's just nothing else you can do.

Former North Carolina Basketball Coach Dean Smith had some words of advice for the die hard types, the Game Seven Guys: "If you make every game a life-and-death thing, you're going to have problems. You'll be dead a lot."

A cousin to the Coach on the Floor is the "Referee on the Floor." This guy can spot a moving pick from fifty feet away. A blade of grass that hangs just over the concrete court is out of bounds. Our Referee on the Floor is Greg Van Dulman, without a doubt.

Greg has called more moving screens on me than I received in my entire career of middle and high school basketball. If a rule is in Greg's NCAA Official Rulebook [which he actually owns], he knows the rule frontward and backward—bylaws included. And he will call it. He'll anticipate it happening and be on the lookout for it. In the history of every pick-up basketball game ever played, only twelve three-second calls have been made [not an official stat], and Greg has called eleven of them [also unofficial].

"We'll argue calls from time to time" Wayne said. "And Greg has even brought his rule book with him a couple times."

"Once the guys said that we were playing by college rules, that's all I needed to hear," Greg said. "I went right down and got the rule book."

Greg admitted he tends to officiate more than some others out on the court but offered a bit of an explanation into his attention to the rules. When he was in high school, he had a physical education teacher who was a fanatic about two things—he taught *physical education*, not gym class and the other thing was basketball.

"He would teach us all of the rules of basketball, and we played basketball all the time," Greg remembered. "We played against each other and he even made us referee the games. That's part of where I got my attention to the rules from."

Greg also used to play basketball during lunch breaks from his job in downtown Cincinnati. During those basketball games at the YMCA, Greg played with guys who had played collegiate basketball. He also played with a guy who had been a college basketball official. He called fouls in the pick-up games just as he had while officiating college games.

"I learned a lot from him about the rules of the game," Greg said. "He called a lot of fouls, but it kept the games civil and that's what I'm trying to do out there on Fran's court. When you've got guys dipping their shoulders down and doing a lot of offensive charging, it ruins the game."

A couple of other stereotype guys: "The Mr. Clean Guy"—the guy who hustles like crazy, not afraid to get on the ground to mop the floor in an attempt to get a loose ball. Jason fits into this category as well as Byron White, Matt Roberts, and Greg Aerni. If Byron is in a pile, he's coming away with the ball.

Greg Aerni is a holiday explosion. When Christmas or Thanksgiving or Easter comes around, you know a visit from Greg might be coming soon. We both look forward to it and cringe at the thought of his athleticism. He is all over the floor—an incredible leaper and a much better athlete than anyone else on that court. He jumps over all of us and never slows, never tires. Fortunately for us [and our collective self-esteem], he doesn't come around too often.

I've known Matt since we were in middle school together. He recently moved to Cincinnati and began playing on Thursday nights with us. He probably fits equally into the Game Seven Guy category and The Mr. Clean group. He is intense and hustles more than anyone I have ever played with or against. On Thursday nights, he relishes the opportunity to trap a ball handler on the baseline, and he will slap the floor in excitement at forcing a turnover. He has always been this way. I have never seen him confront any situation at anything less than full throttle. It has been fun to reconnect with Matt after all these years and play basketball with him like we once did when we were kids.

Another group would be the "Garbage Men." These are the guys that turn our bad shots into put backs. They clean up clanks and bricks and keep offensive possessions alive all night long. Wayne belongs in this group and so did former player Ken Ohnemus. Ken lives in Seattle now, but anytime he is in the same time zone as Cincinnati, you can be sure Ken and his left-handed jumper will find his way to the brightly lit court on Apple Ridge Lane. Fran remembered Ken as a hustler, one who was always on the boards in the right place at the right time. Mike Brunner, one of the original players, also belonged in this group before a nasty injury ended his playing days.

"He was just incredible at getting rebounds for stick backs," Fran said of Mike. "He was just awesome. He would always find a way to be exactly where he needed to be to get a rebound and get a stick back. He didn't jump high, but he just had a way of positioning himself.

"Wayne does a lot of rebounding, but he's just out there skying and cutting across the lane," Fran continued. "Mike just knew where the ball was coming off; he'd get there and he was very quick. The ball never hit the floor. It would hit his hands and it'd be back off the backboard and in."

We also have "The Gunners." These guys haven't met a shot they don't like. Fran fits into this category [I can fit into this category, depending on the night]. But, perhaps our most prolific Gunner is Byron Heizer.

If feet are planted squarely on anything resembling a basketball court, Byron, dressed head-to-toe in Ohio State gear, thinks [and is often correct] he is within range. When his back isn't acting up on him, Byron can get in a groove unlike any of us. When he gets on a run, he'll shoot ten times a game. The rest of the guys will just defer to him and step back for long rebounds because if he does miss, that ball is going to careen some twenty or so feet. I've seen him make six consecutive threes to close out a [quick] game to twenty. He'll be falling into the grass and the shot will still go down.

Alas, the law of averages is the greatest villain to our Gunners. But we adhere to a certain motto to get us through droughts: "The best way to get out of a shooting slump is to shoot your way out."

And then there are the "Magic Johnson Guys"—when you are on a team with these guys, you better have your eyes on the ball because a no-look pass is certain to be heading your way, usually nose high. We've got a trio of these guys—Greg Van Dulman, John Orr, and Jerry Moore, who, a few years ago, hung up his high tops for good because of nagging injuries.

"Jerry had a way of passing the ball that was like some kind of no-look pass that was on a B-line," Fran remembered. "It got to the point where I went out and bought a mouth guard just to guard against Jerry Moore's passes. He doesn't play anymore, so I've never had to use it."

There are a couple of guarantees on the court: John seemingly will always make his first shot of the night, Wayne will hit a gamer, and Fran will surprise a newcomer [or even some of the regulars] when he takes and makes a thirty-foot three-pointer to win a game.

"You gotta get out on him," I'll yell.

"He was thirty feet from the basket!" will be the defender's argument.

"I know where he was!"

I've been on the receiving end of that shot more than enough times in the decade I've known Fran to give him more than an inch on any shot. I'll guard him at the base of the driveway if I have to. Come to think of it, I think I have.

It's fun to play against the same guys for years and understand how they play and what they'll do in certain situations. It makes the competition tighter. It forces us to come up with something new; it forces us to adjust. It makes us better. It's what differentiates our game from a pick-up game on some indiscriminate court against random players.

We all have signature plays.

John has a spinning scoop shot in the lane, one in which he always seems to go the opposite direction his defender expects. He's also deadly on his first shot of the night. I honestly cannot remember the last time John missed his first shot.

Greg Van Dulman, whose defensive lineman frame comes with just a bit more padding these days, has a semi-backward set shot that he makes with incredible proficiency in the lane. He'll back you into the lane and, when the opportunity calls for a turnaround jumper, he'll twist just enough to see the rim before sinking the set shot. He, too, can get on quite a three-pointer run from time to time. He hops into his jumpers from a semi-crouched position, a shot Jerry Moore referred to as a *froggy shot*. He's definitely one of our better shooters. You do not leave him unguarded.

"Defense was always my strength growing up," Greg said. "But when you get old and you can't play defense anymore, you better learn to shoot."

Roger brings the Kareem sky hook that is impossible to block. He can be triple teamed and it doesn't matter—that shot is going up and that shot is going in. He'll carry a team from time to time on that shot alone.

Fran's dazzling reverse lay-ups have given all of us fits. You know it's coming, too. You try to force him to the baseline, but he'll wriggle into the perfect spot and spin the ball off the backboard like a billiard star smacking the cue ball with just the right amount of English.

Jason's three-point—wait, his foot was on the line again—shot is a nightly occurrence. If Jason was a superhero, and I'm not saying he's not, the three-point line would be his kryptonite. I wonder how many almost game winners Jason has made when his team had seventeen points only to be awarded just the two because the tip of his toe was on the line. With every shot, "on the line!" or "that's a two!" can be heard from one of the relieved defenders.

Jason also brings an intensity to the court. He is calm and collected off of the court, a man driven by proper perspective and the Golden Rule. On the court, especially on the defensive end, he is a mad man [he once even mistakenly ripped the ball out of a teammate's arms]. He does not like to give the offensive player an inch of breathing room, especially after giving up an open shot on a previous play. He rarely leaves anything on the court.

"It's awesome to wake up Friday morning groggy and short of sleep, sore and achy, and unable to even trot until loosened up," he said. "These ails only remind me that I'm alive, and that I truly gave my all the night before."

Byron White, strong and athletic like a shorter Karl Malone, has a unique jump shot. He gets just high enough to not get the shot blocked—the ball itself has backspin similar to a Tiger Woods chip shot. The ball hits the back of the rim and almost stops. There is no bounce and usually, that ball slowly crawls through the hoop.

Byron's son, Kevin, has recently become a regular with our group. He is entertaining to watch. His athleticism trumps all of ours. It has been fun to include him in the group. I finally get to see what it is like to play against someone a decade younger than me. I've noticed some of the older guys play really hard when they are guarding me and I've noticed that my effort level increases when I play against Kevin. There's something inside that kicks in and forces you to show the young guy that you can still play with him. Kevin is deadly in the paint; his rebounding and ability to finish inside is indefensible. If his shot is on, he is unbeatable.

Wayne's signature move may have nothing to do with taking a shot. His would be his ability to rebound, especially when his team is on the offensive end. He has kept more possessions alive than anyone on that court; it's such a relief to have him on your team, knowing he will clean up your mess. When Wayne is on my team, I shoot more because I know that if I miss, he'll be there to pick me up.

As far as shots are concerned, though, Wayne's signature shot would have to be his late night game-winners from about fifteen feet away. When the game is on the line, defenders pack the paint and refuse to surrender a layup. That doesn't stop most of us from driving the lane for a finisher. But when Wayne is on my team and we are two points from a win, I will drive the lane but with no intent whatsoever of shooting. I know Wayne is out there floating around the foul line or the wing waiting. I'll drive, find Wayne, and get him the ball any way I can. Once the ball is in his hands in that particular situation, I'll start heading over to my water bottle because I am certain his shot is going down.

Byron Heizer's fall-away three-pointers are something to behold. There have been times where I'll anticipate his fall away and lean in to get my hand closer to the ball. No matter. I can be right on him, and it doesn't bother him when he's on his game.

We may all be a little different on the court, but one thing that we all bring with us on Thursday nights is a bit of passion and energy. These games are not walks in the park. We all want to win; some more than others, but the effort is far beyond simply respectable.

"All the guys are quite competitive," Jason said. "We really, really want to win every point and every game. However, when the game's over, there's nothing but graciousness and goodness. [We have] a very good group of guys that I personally believe God had a role in placing together."

When grandpas are on the court diving for loose balls or stifling a good shooter's shot with suffocating defense, you can't help but be inspired out there. We've got guys who'll admit they're not in the best of shape, but who go all out when they are on the court. There may be games when the shots just won't fall, but rarely—if ever—do you see a game when the regular players aren't giving everything they've got.

It's fun to see some newcomers on Thursday and, when seeing the older or the *experienced* group—as they like to be called—expect a different type of game.

"Some of my favorite memories," Jason said, "are when young guys occasionally show up cocky and leave humbled."

One of those young guys—although he's never been one to appear cocky—is Luke Howell, Roger's college-aged son. He grew up wanting to go watch his dad play on Thursdays when Roger played with a different group, sometimes attending as a kid when his mother was away. He and his brother, Wes, would sit on the gymnasium stage and watch the games, noticing the joy that each of the players seemed to have splashed all over their faces.

By the time Luke was in high school, he would ask his dad if he could come and play on Thursdays with our group.

"No," Roger told him. "You're too young."

Luke wanted just one game to see what it would be like and to see how well the guys could play. Roger kept telling Luke that he was too fast and too energetic to play. Once during the summer after Luke graduated from high school, his dad invited him to play one Thursday night because attendance would be a little low.

"I just ran around like I usually played and was a little too crazy for the group," Luke said, who admitted he's more of a baseball guy than a basketball player. "I didn't play again for a few years. So my dad was kind of correct. It took a few years of maturity and another chance on a slow day for me to actually get it right."

He has more than gotten it right since he became a regular during summers and holiday breaks away from the University of Kentucky. Luke is lightning in a bottle. Where he once seemed out of control, he has learned to harness his bursts and has become one of the better players out on the court. He has developed a devastating baby hook shot in the lane, undoubtedly something he picked up from watching his old man all of these years.

Luke has learned a lot from Roger, who has served as Luke's mentor and coach for most of his childhood. The learning has not waned.

"I have really enjoyed sharing this experience with my dad, especially because he's the one that I learn the most from," Luke said. "He has coached me in a variety of sports throughout my life, and he will always be my coach. It's nice to continue to learn from him. Driving home, we always go over that night's games and that's where I learn what he likes and what he doesn't. Overall, it's always fun to play with him, interesting to play against him, and it's great to be able share playing basketball with him every week."

Luke said that, being young, he felt he would have an advantage out on the Thursday night court because of the ages of those against whom he would be playing.

"I had played basketball enough with my dad to know that he could shoot, and so I assumed that most of the other guys could shoot as well," he said. "Which, I was totally correct about. However, I was expecting it to be slow paced with a lot of screens, post-ups, and jumpers."

What he didn't expect was the speed of the game. The guys that show up on Thursdays do a pretty good job of keeping themselves in shape, or they wouldn't even bother showing up. To this day, I'm still in awe of how those who are in their fifties and sixties play the game. They may have lost a step or two, but if you don't bring your best against them, you will be humbled.

"The first few times that I came, I would not go at a 100 percent; I didn't want to hurt anyone or be that annoying young kid that ran all over the place," Luke said. "However, as I became more comfortable and started having to guard people like Aaron and Jason more, I realized that even if I tried my hardest, they were going to score on me with their annoying jumpers, so I needed to guard them my hardest and try to limit the damage. Even some of the older guys like Fran and Wayne move so much quicker than they should for their age; it's still a workout to keep up with them."

I hate to break it to Luke; he *is* that annoying young kid running all over the place; he's just learned how to play the game the right way, which makes him all the more annoying.

FAMILY GUYS

In 2013, Valentine's Day fell on a Thursday. I woke up bright and early and saw this e-mail from Jason that was sent to all of the Thursday night crew.

> Valentine's day? Yes, Valentine's day. But isn't it only right to celebrate properly on a Friday or Saturday with your beloved?? Who's in for hoops?

Valentine's Day, birthdays, and anniversaries that fall on Thursday nights can be tricky waters to navigate. Fortunately for me, my father-in-law had been working on my excuse long before I was even in the picture.

"Lucky for you that Chrissy was brought up with this, so you didn't have to break her in," Fran told me. "It's never been too uncomfortable around our house anyway when it comes to birthdays and anniversaries. Peg knows that everybody's going to be outside, and I need to go out. So, whether it's her fiftieth birthday or our twenty-fifth wedding anniversary, I can't remember ever missing a Thursday night hoop game for anything like that."

It's that mentality that Chrissy grew up with, so I don't need to really plead my case on Thursdays, no matter the occasion. Thanks a lot for that, Fran!

But not all of us are willing to postpone an important night with our significant other because of basketball.

"I'm not stupid," Mike Brunner said without hesitation.

One Thursday evening, Jason's parents were in town and invited his three daughters to spend the night with them, leaving Jason home alone with his wife, Sherry. Jason is a regular for a reason; he is committed to our game and he showed up to play that night.

"That may not have been the best decision I've ever made," he admitted with a smile. If Jason has to take a Thursday off in the near future, we'll understand. Most of us will, anyway.

Some of the wives, though, come to depend on basketball night as much as the guys. Amy Orr, John's wife, has come to rely on his participation in Thursday night basketball. One particular Thursday evening, Amy went out with a friend to enjoy a movie and then she returned home for a quiet evening to herself. Visions of peace and a quiet night of reading filled her head. She parked the car, entered the home, and then, "What are you doing here?"

John had taken the night off. It was supposed to rain that night [it didn't] and John had decided to give his body a needed break. Amy wasn't mentally prepared for that audible.

"I think she needs Thursday nights as much as I do," John said, laughing. "She makes plans on Thursday night and they do not include me."

Most of the men in this group are married and many have children, some young and some grown. We all have responsibilities to our families, whether it is driving sons and daughters to college or attempting to get them to bed before we leave for basketball on Thursday nights. We are all busy with work or volunteering and free nights with families come preciously too seldom. But a night on the court is just as important to our health and well-being as spending a night at home. And, for the most part, the wives would agree.

"My wife is very supportive of my playing," Wayne said. "Maybe it's because I don't get much exercise, and she wants me to get some. Maybe it's because she gets me out of the house and has time to herself. Maybe it's because she knows I won't be seeking sex that night! Who knows? But she understands that on Thursdays, I'm gone."

Roger's wife is equally as supportive.

"Kathy is almost as committed to Thursday night hoops as I am," Roger said. "She knows I need the exercise and the stress relief. She knows it has to be a major reason for me to miss. She is amazing."

But what about birthdays and anniversaries?

"We are usually on vacation in August during her birthday and our anniversary," Roger said. "So, fortunately it has not been an issue. Seems like good planning to me."

Well played, Roger.

Pat Hanlon understood the unwritten law in his house: if there was work to get done, it best be done by Thursday night.

"Other than my family, Thursday night basketball is the most satisfying thing I was ever a part of," Pat said. "It was just something you really look forward to. If you had some work to do at home, you wanted to get it done before Thursday night so the old lady wouldn't bug you about playing basketball."

Getting us out of the house means one thing to our wives, but certainly another thing to our young children.

I remember when my oldest daughter, Sierra, was around two or three, she would be sad when she saw me getting dressed into my basketball clothes after dinner. She would be in tears and give me a hug and not want me to leave. It was hard to leave her.

Things have changed.

Now, she knows it's Thursday night long before I get my high-tops out of the closet. My five-year-old son asks me on Tuesday if I'm going to play basketball with grandpa. When I say no, he responds with a disappointed, "Oh, man."

They look forward to "mommy time" when I'm gone. They know that when I'm home, bedtime is bedtime. But when I'm not there, bedtime can be negotiated.

"Mommy, since Daddy's playing basketball tonight, can we watch a movie?" Sierra will whisper thinking I am out of earshot.

Or, less subtly, she'll yell, "Yay! Snuggle Night!" On these nights, I'll return from basketball and find children sleeping in any number of beds and rooms in our house. Sometimes, Chrissy will be asleep on the couch with one of the kids next to her. Sometimes, the four of them will be crammed onto one full-sized mattress, complete with arms and legs dangling over the edge.

One evening, my wife and I had miraculously convinced each of our three children to lie in their own beds. Each promised to go to sleep. However, bedtime promises are as flimsy as a suspension bridge made of balsa wood.

I headed toward the door leading to the garage, opened it, and then closed it again without going through it just to see what would happen. Less than five seconds after the sound of the door closing, my daughter sprinted out into the living room with a huge smile on her face that quickly dissipated the moment she noticed I hadn't left. I just smiled at her and let Chrissy deal with bedtime that night.

Mike Kraine has had similar struggles leaving his house on Thursday nights.

"My wife, she doesn't seem to mind," Mike said. "I just tell her it's keeping me from getting fat, and she says, 'Okay.' The kids, though, get really upset and cry. They hang on my legs, begging me not to go. They usually fall off at the garage door threshold. It kind of tears me up when they do that, but what can you do? It's basketball."

Basketball has a way of pushing the reset button. It clears and cleans the mind of frustrations and stresses. There will be nights when I'm upset at one of my kids or just frustrated with something at home. I'll go and play three hours of basketball, and when I return home, for me, there seems to have been some sort of detox of the mind. I walk around the quiet house and put all the kids back in their own beds. Each one looks like an angel. I'm not mad anymore. I'm not frustrated. I'm not stressed.

Everything seemingly is perfect again.

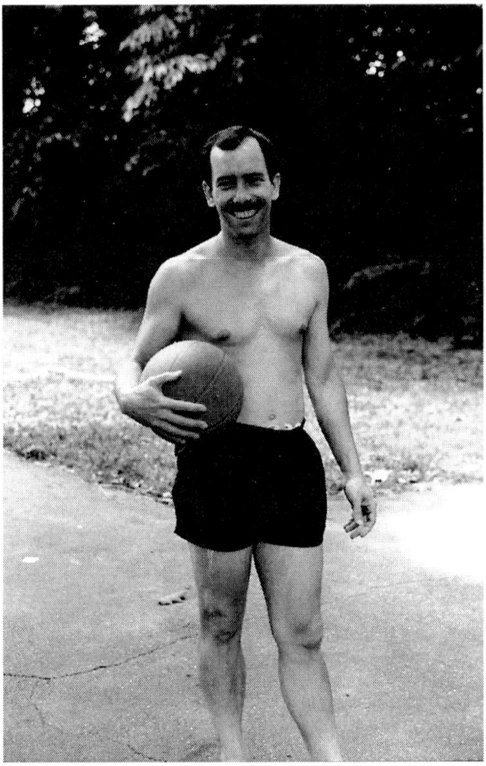

Fran Niehaus stands on his very own Court of Dreams in the summer of 1985.

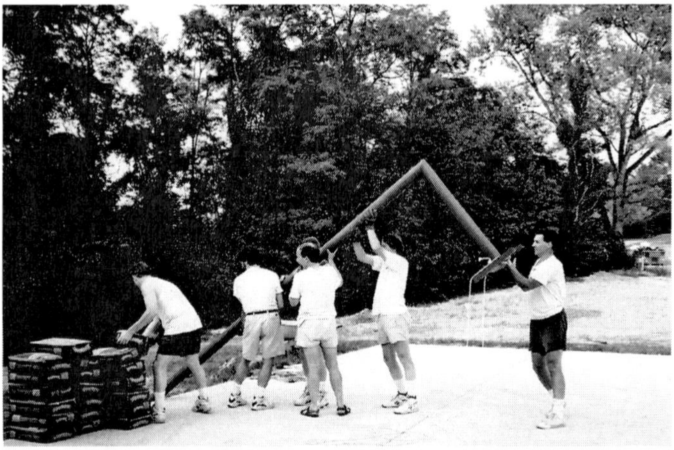

In 1993, Fran Niehaus moved to Apple Ridge Lane where he built his Court of Dreams 2.0. The guys begin to lay the cement foundation for the basketball pole.

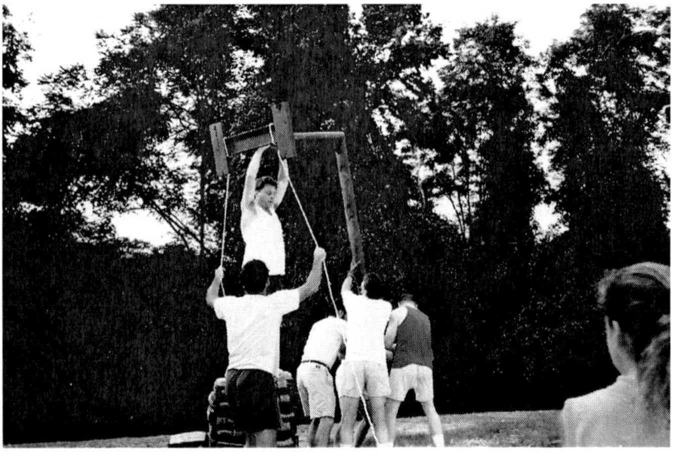

Greg Van Dulman helps steady the pole as the guys help build Fran's new court.

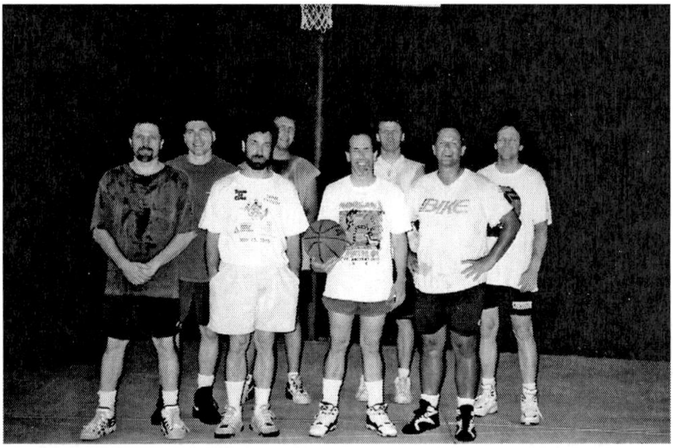

(Back) Ken Ohnemus, Terry Fazenbacher, Paul Smith, Wayne Jones (Front) Greg Van Dulman, Fred Miller, Fran Niehaus, "Shooting Dan" Furlong pose on the court in 1997.

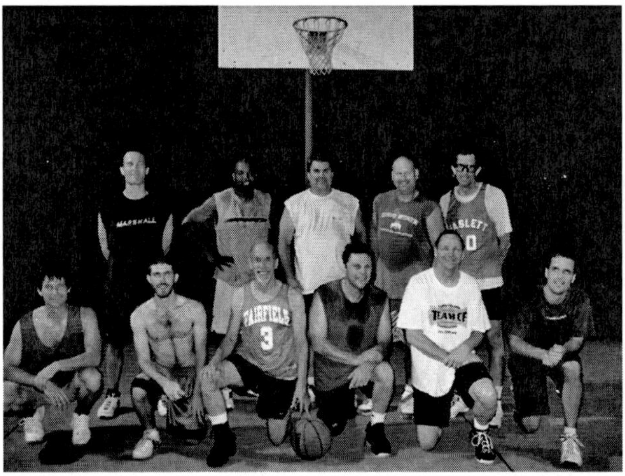

(Back) Mike Kraine, Byron White, John Orr, Byron Heizer, Roger Howell (Front) Scott Gordon, Sam Lieberman, Fran Niehaus, Greg Van Dulman, Wayne Jones, Jason Angelo pose on Fran's court in 2006.

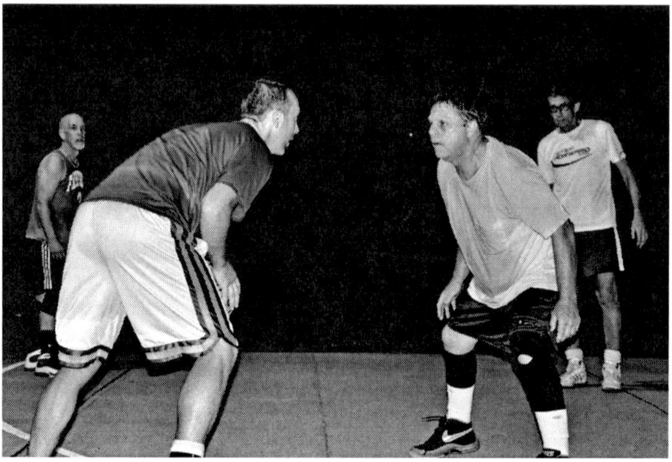

Greg Van Dulman stares down Aaron Smith on the court.

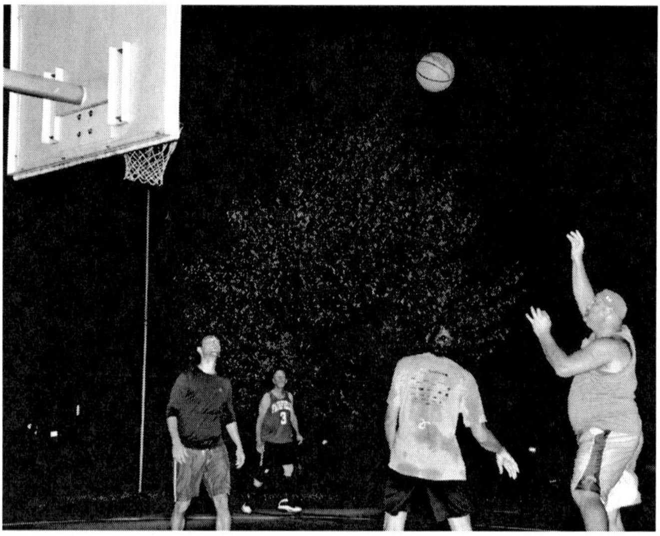

Byron Heizer lofts a short jumper in the
lane as Roger Howell defends.

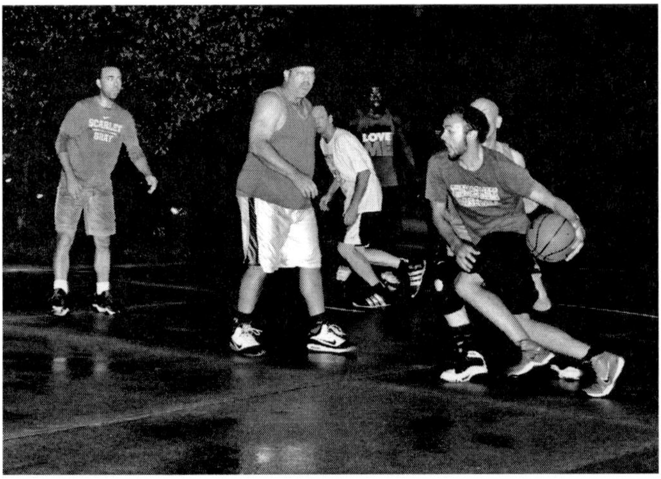

Luke Howell, Roger's son, drives past the defense on his way for another two points in the lane.

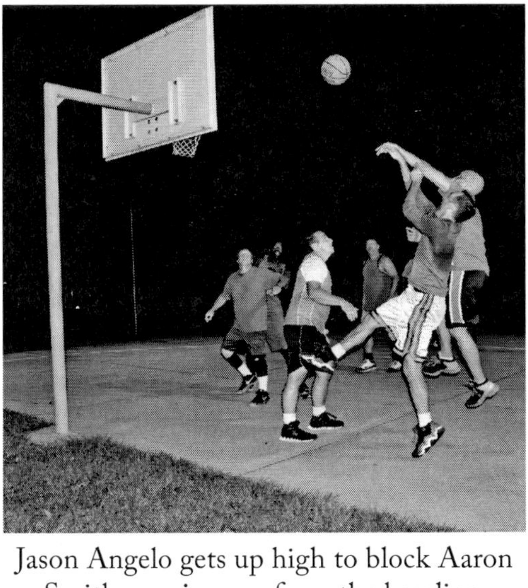

Jason Angelo gets up high to block Aaron Smith on a jumper from the baseline.

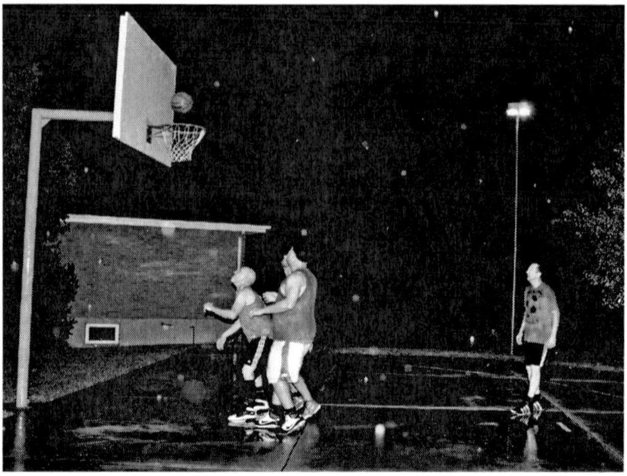

Rain doesn't usually put a damper on Thursday Night basketball. When it does, it has to rain a lot harder than this.

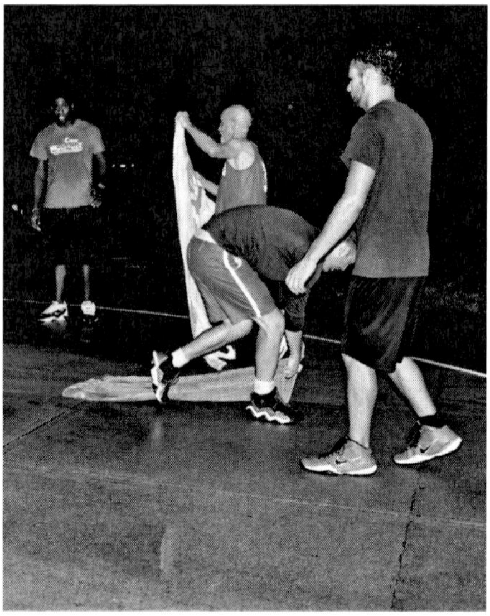

Aaron Smith and Fran Niehaus towel off the rain puddles between games.

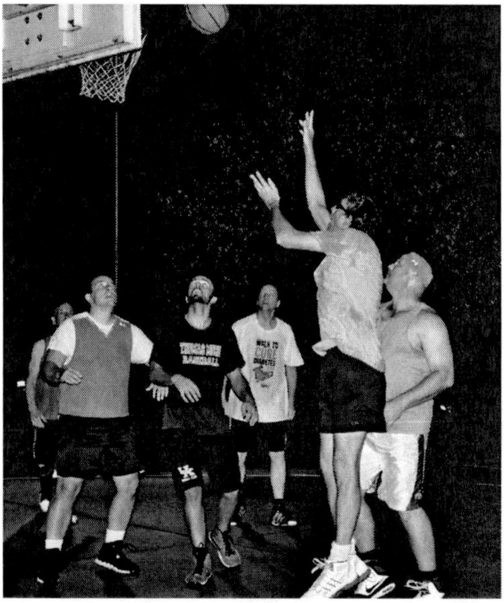

Roger Howell is a dominating force inside.

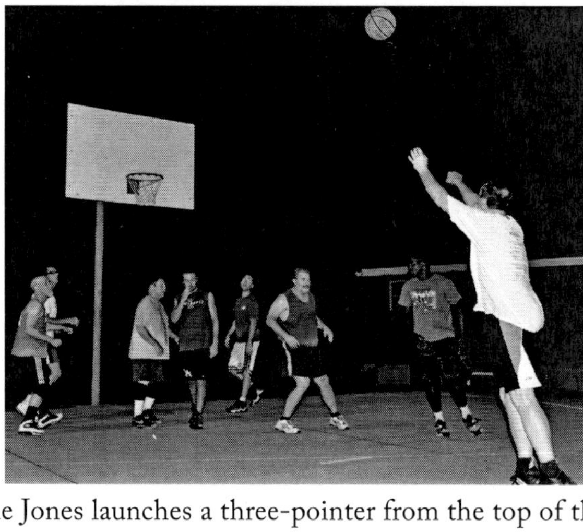

Wayne Jones launches a three-pointer from the top of the key.

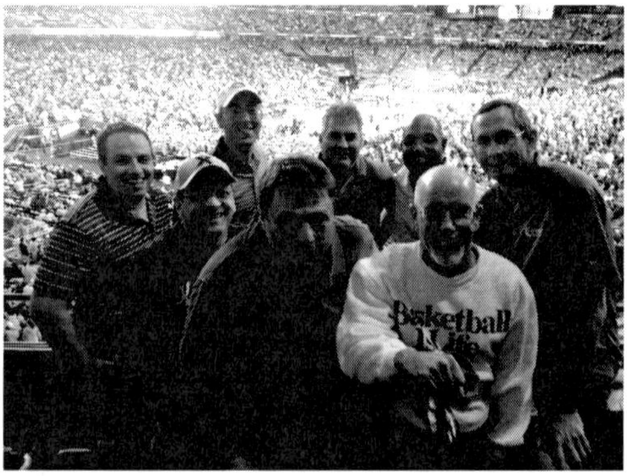

(Back) Matt Roberts, Aaron Smith, John Orr, Byron White, Roger Howell (Front) Wayne Jones, Greg Van Dulman, Fran Niehaus attend the NCAA Championship Game in Atlanta in 2013.

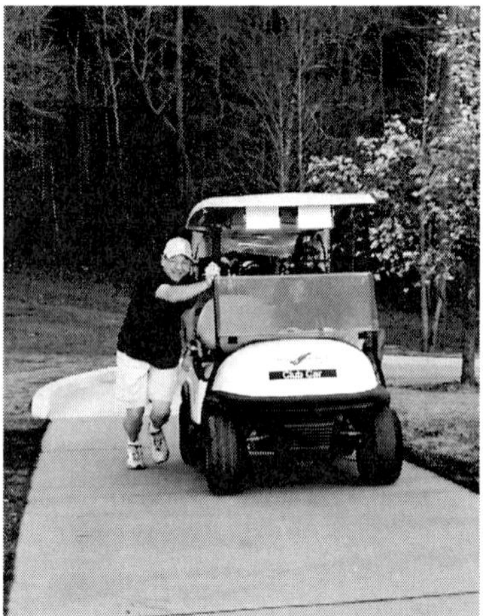

While in Georgia for the Final Four and a trip to the Masters practice round, the guys got in a couple rounds of golf. Here, Wayne Jones pushes while Byron White steers the golf cart, which lost all battery power, up a hill at Cherokee Run Golf Course in Conyers, GA.

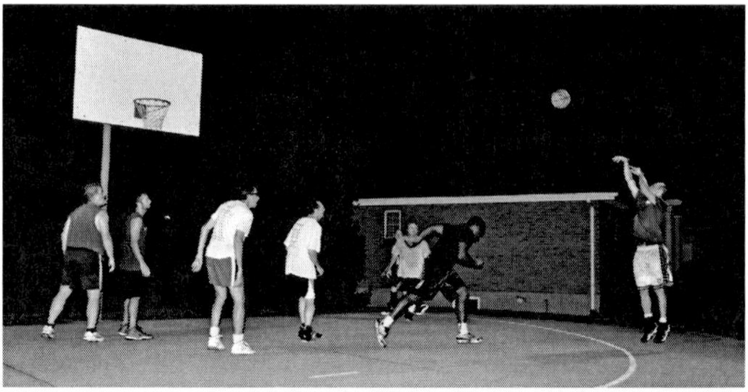

Aaron Smith fires up a three-pointer as
Kevin White charges on defense.

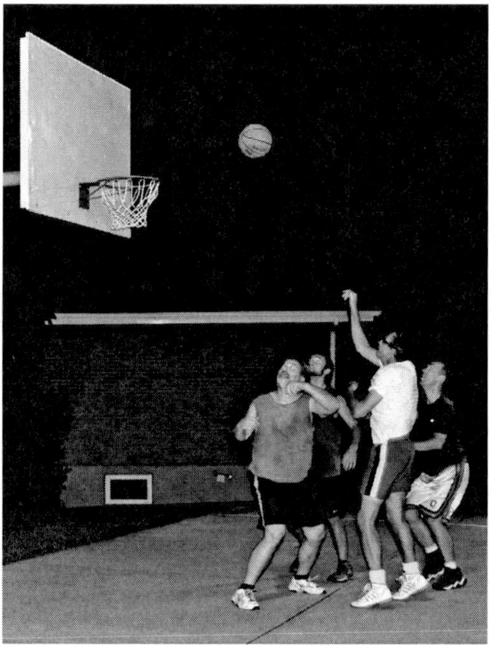

Roger Howell is unfazed by the traffic in the lane.

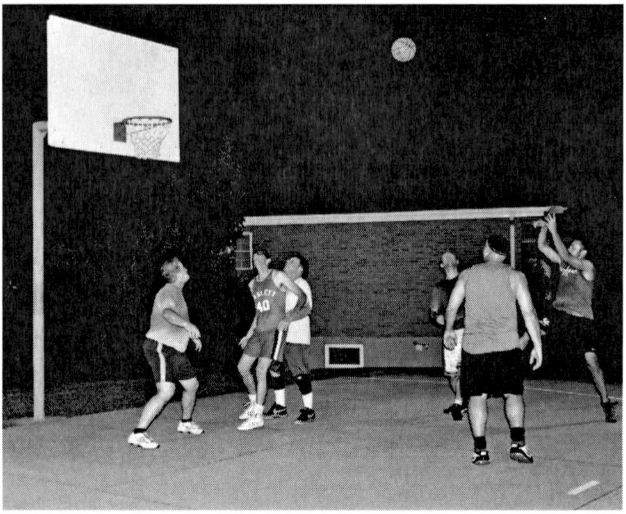

Luke Howell shoots a fade-away, knowing his dad
Roger (#40) will grab the rebound if he misses.

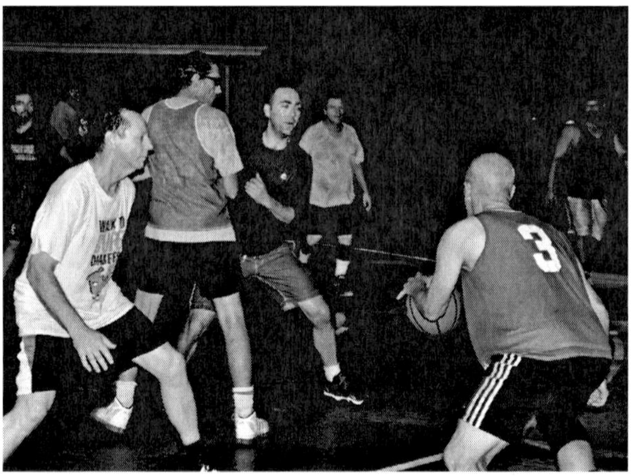

Fran Niehaus tries to read the defense as Roger Howell sets
the pick on Aaron Smith while Wayne Jones defends.

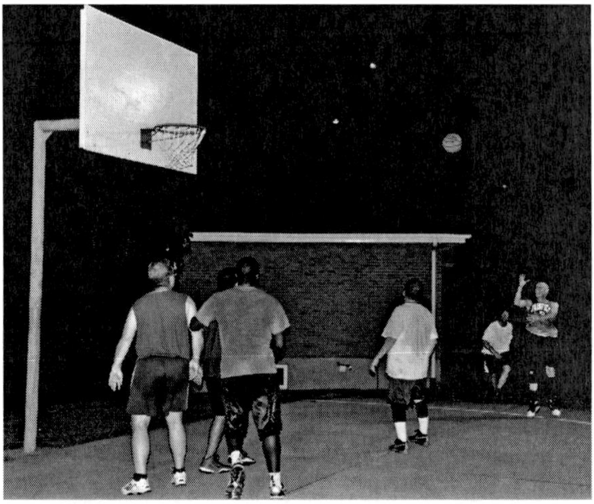

Fran Niehaus is automatic from three-point range.

Wayne Jones is known for his game-winners. Here, he sets up in his favorite spot ready to hit another gamer.

CAMARADERIE ON AND OFF THE COURT

> In basketball, as in life, true joy comes from being fully present in each and every moment.
>
> —Phil Jackson

It was about nine in the evening on a warm Thursday, and I was running a little late. I had just spent the last ninety minutes trying to convince three young children that it was bedtime and that, "No, it's not snuggle night." There had been tears and screaming and pleading—mostly from the kids. I just wanted to get to Fran's house. Three miles and change were all that rested between insanity and emergency therapy.

I performed one final bed check. My oldest daughter and my son had given up the good fight. They were finally asleep, sprawled sideways on their mattresses like prize fighters knocked unconscious for the first time. My youngest daughter clung to my wife as the two of them lay next to each other in a warm comfortable ball in the middle of our bed. I inhaled deeply and shut my eyes. At long last.

I had been in my basketball armor since seven o'clock; the countdown began, though, an hour before that. Once dinner was scraped from our dining table and dishes hastily stuffed into the dishwasher and trash cans thrown to the curb, I was ready to prepare for the night of basketball that had been beckoning like a Siren's enchanting call.

I get ready for basketball the way my wife gets ready for work or a night out. First, I had to find the right outfit—um, I mean uniform. Was it hot? Cold? Windy? It all mattered. Shorts or sweatpants? Long sleeve or short sleeve? Thermal? Did I need to bring a towel in case of high humidity? Have I had good shooting nights in this shirt or not? Did my shoes match my shirt? Okay, that last one wasn't exactly accurate, but point made.

Which braces did I need that night? Ankle? Check. Knee? Nah. Finger? Probably should, but not going to. Shoulder? Not that night; it messed with my shot. Wrist? Why did I even own that brace?

Once I figured out what to wear, I turned my attention to my feet. One pair of socks—the long ones. Then a second pair—ankle length. Then, I strapped a brace on my right foot that still felt the effects of a ruptured Achilles tendon suffered four years prior. Finally, I yanked on my Adidas high tops and tied a double knot.

Next, I filled a large jug with ice water and downed some multi-vitamins. And just before I could finally leave, I dug in the medicine cabinet and premedicated myself with a couple Advils and a glass of milk. I was finally ready.

It was game time! One of these days, I'm going to get a speeding ticket on my way to Fran's on Thursday night. But that Thursday was not that night.

I turned left onto Apple Ridge Lane and could see the glow. I rounded the curve and proceeded down the hill. The lights high atop the garage were splashing the dusk summer sky like the lights that illuminated Ray Kinsella's baseball field the night he and Terrence Mann returned to Iowa from Minnesota. On the near side of the basketball court was a group of four, maybe five guys raising a seventeen-foot-high light post. Silhouetted by the garage lights behind them, they resembled the American soldiers at Iwo Jima, raising the beautiful Stars and Stripes atop Mount Suribachi during World War II.

I pulled off the side of the street behind a couple of cars. I took off my glasses and put on a pair of old glasses that miraculously still existed after several years of being elbowed and slapped to the concrete [Note: I have since gone to contacts. All pairs of old glasses have been destroyed on the court]. I grabbed my red and white reversible jersey and my water and trudged up the driveway, tired from a long day.

"Good to see you," one of the group said. "You're our eighth. Time to go fours!"

"Shoot 'em up," Fran said.

The first four who made free throws were on one team and those who did not make free throws were on the other. Sometimes, when our free-throw shooting would resemble a series of Shaquille O'Neal free-throw attempts, someone could be heard shouting, "Layup line!" We never do shoot layups, though. We are stubborn. We'll keep on shooting until we have what we need. That is the rule.

Just getting to Fran's house on time is the first wave of adrenaline on Thursday nights for many of us. The time we have to spend with each other is paramount to our well-being and much effort goes in to being there. We feel a responsibility to be there, not just for our own physical and mental needs, but for the others that we know will show up. We count on each other to be there every Thursday night so we can have enough to play.

"Thursday night hoops has brought me many a good friend," Wayne said. "It has also allowed me to do something I love for many, many years. It's filled my need for male companionship, exercise, and competition. It's given me support for the trials I've faced in life. It's given me friends, some of whom are like a second family."

SECOND FAMILY

For a while, one of our regular players, John Orr, would spend the night in Cincinnati on Thursday nights because of our regular game. He and his wife Amy lived in Kentucky at the time, and from their home, it was about an hour commute to his office in Cincinnati. On Thursdays, he would work and then stay in Cincinnati until it was time to head to Fran's house for basketball.

There he would run, cut, shoot, and rebound, burning the stresses of the week off with every step toward the basket. By 11:30 or midnight, after the last shot of the night had fallen through the net, John would drive to his wife's parents' house and spend the night there instead of going all the way back home. He would then go to work on Friday before returning home that night.

"I didn't do that a ton, but for about a year or so, yeah, I would sleep over at the in-laws after basketball," John said. "That may give you some sense of my commitment to the game."

Roger Howell, a smart ball player with a swimmer's body, began playing with Fran's group about two decades ago. For a while, he coached swimming and then raced home on Thursday nights. There was just enough time for him to scarf down dinner, change, and then get on the road to Apple Ridge.

"Now," he said, "I try to eat around 7 o'clock and then take my vitamins before I leave. I get there in time to warm up a few minutes, and then I'm ready to go."

Roger, now in his fifties, said that going through that effort to get to the basketball game is worth it because of what Thursday night hoops does for him.

"It is great exercise, and it relieves stress," he said. "There are friendships. I feel better and am happier. Plus, it keeps my body young and healthy."

No matter how one gets there, all can attest to the need to be there. This Thursday night game needs to exist for each of us in one form or another. Perhaps Wayne put it best.

"You really begin to look forward to Thursday night," he said. "You clear your schedule, get things out of the way, and plan your week around it. On nights of questionable weather, Fran calls people to make sure we can get enough to play.

"Fran has been the glue that keeps this going all these years," Wayne continued. "His love for the game draws others to be part of it. He brings us together for parties at his house, for golf outings, and trips to the Final Four. He allows us to use his place for the game, even when he's on vacation. He provides the court, the balls, and nets and just asks us to make the trip out. Fran has become a great friend for life, both on the court and off. I've been fortunate to have met him and to have been able to be a part of Thursday night hoops."

For one of Fran's barbecues, he invited all of our families. It was good for them to see the people we were hanging out with every Thursday night.

"At first, Sherry thought it was a bit nutty and obsessive about how devoted I was to attending each Thursday," Jason said about his wife. "It seemed to her that it was interfering with 'our' time a bit too much. However, Fran once hosted a cookout at his house for spouses and families. That changed everything. She saw that it wasn't simply about running around and putting a ball in a hoop; she saw the quality and character of the guys and has never since thought of it as frivolous or nonessential."

Fran also provides a valuable service on those Thursday nights that feature big games on television. When the NBA Finals are on television or the World Series, Fran will go inside his house and move his entire television set so that it faces the court through the living room window. We'll all gather around during breaks between our games to "see how the pros do it."

"There are games that I personally would have never seen but for the fact that they were on Thursday night," Fran said. "That World Series game [Game 6 of St. Louis Cardinals vs. Texas Rangers in 2011—a most incredible game] was on a Thursday. I would never have been up to watch that if we weren't watching it on Thursday night. That was a whale of a game. The best was when we used to play outdoors all year round and March Madness was on Thursday nights. That was always very special."

As Wayne mentioned, this group doesn't simply just get together on Thursdays for a night of basketball. There's more to it. We gathered at Fran's house for a party to celebrate the group's twentieth anniversary of playing basketball back in 2004. Fran once had someone film the group playing basketball years ago from a tree on the property.

"I especially remember [Fran's] brother Greg's alley-oop pass to me," Wayne said about the video. "If I could jump, I would have slammed it home. But because I can't, I had to lay it in off the glass, but it still looked pretty good on tape."

Many of us gathered at a surprise birthday party for Wayne—these guys are more than just warm bodies on a basketball court.

"These are special people and I have a lot of respect for them," Greg Van Dulman said. "It was great to go to Wayne's party and sit around a table and talk to the guys, seeing what's going on in their lives outside of basketball. Basketball is our focal point, but it's the guys that bring us back every week."

Each year, we get the whole group together for at least one round of golf—getting to know each other off of the basketball court has been refreshing and enjoyable for many of us.

"I took up playing golf with these guys because I know that there will be a day when I won't be able to play basketball with them anymore," Greg said. "It will hurt when I won't be able to play basketball anymore, but at least I'll have golf and I'll still get to spend time with the guys."

And, every few years or so, we all get together for a trip to the Final Four when it comes to Indianapolis, Detroit, or Atlanta. The best is when the Final Four is in Atlanta. The Masters Tournament in Augusta is also played the following week and is just a short few hours away.

Consider the trip a sort of sports pilgrimage.

In 2013, the stars aligned once again as the Final Four was scheduled for the Georgia Dome in Atlanta. The basketball games were Saturday and Monday; the days between were for golfing. We left for Atlanta on Friday morning; we could have left Thursday, but we all were otherwise occupied.

Sore and tight from the previous night's round of basketball, we climbed into various minivans and headed due south for a sports weekend of a lifetime. We stopped on the way down in Knoxville, Tennessee, for a round of golf at Dead Horse Lake Golf Course.

I had been placed in charge of picking out the golf courses, and I found Dead Horse Lake after a Google search. The website had gorgeous pictures of a rolling landscape with an emerald green course. It had been voted east Tennessee's best public golf course. My heart sank, though, as we pulled into the driveway. Dead Horse Lake indeed. The grass, however, looked far worse off than the unfortunate horse. There was nothing but soggy fields of what looked like closely shorn and matted straw. My only job was to pick golf courses and set up tee times, and the first course we went to looked like it was under construction. It wasn't however, and somehow, we were able to play a round.

The grass was not dead, we later found out. It was simply Bermuda grass that had not yet turned green. We were assured that sometime soon it would be gorgeous. But on that particular day, it was anything but. Once the sloppy round was over, it was time for dinner. And what better place to eat in the South than a quality barbecue joint?

On Saturday, we spent the day in Atlanta, feeling the nervous energy of those wearing Louisville, Wichita State, Syracuse, and Michigan colors. I supported my alma mater and wore my Ohio University Bobcats shirt, feeling no anxiety whatsoever. Inside the Georgia Dome, we watched Louisville stop the Shockers and Michigan thwart the Orangemen. Born in Columbus and a faithful Buckeye fan,

I wasn't sure how I'd be able to handle being in the dome for a Wolverine championship. I suddenly became a huge Louisville supporter.

After the games, we drove about forty-five minutes east to Conyers where we were staying. Some of us stayed up late into the night, talking basketball and enjoying a meal at the local IHOP just across the street from the hotel.

On Sunday, I got my redemption as we went to the spectacular Cherokee Run Golf Club. This stunning course was nestled in the rolling hills within the Georgia International Horse Park. The Arnold Palmer-designed course was dotted with gorgeous pine trees that lined most of the fairways. There were granite outcroppings exploding around many of the greens, creating an unbelievably scenic round of golf. This course was everything Dead Horse Lake was not. Despite several of our carts running out of battery juice and having to be pushed up steep inclines, it was one of the most beautiful rounds of golf most of us had played.

Monday morning was an early one. A five-in-the-morning wake-up call jolted us from our beds and out onto the early-morning road to Augusta for the first practice round of the Master's Tournament. Augusta National Golf Club had been a bucket list item for many of us, so the early start to the day was not an issue.

Despite contradicting GPS devices and a long line of traffic, we found the golf course via a short jaunt through South Carolina and back to Georgia. We parked and took our position in the throng shuffling to Augusta National's gates. Once inside, we were transported to some sort of paradise, one in which the closely cropped grass was mistaken for artificial field turf. Not a single weed was present, not a single blade of grass misplaced. It was spectacular—

an outdoor cathedral. From Amen Corner to the stunning azaleas to the spot on the tenth hole where Bubba Watson hit his mind-blowing and memorable shot in 2012, we strolled the grounds with our jaws dropped in amazement. It truly was a magical experience.

From Augusta National, we raced back to Atlanta in time for the National Championship Game between Louisville and Michigan. The electric atmosphere was a reminder of why we play the game; the skill displayed was an inspiration to each of us. After watching Louisville win late and cut down the championship nets, all we wanted to do was get to Thursday so we could try our best to impersonate the best.

The trip was memorable; we got to spend time with each other in a different way. Playing and watching golf was a great opportunity to get to know each other off of the basketball court, but basketball is the glue that holds this group together.

"We've had hundreds of players over the years and mostly all of them were great guys," Wayne said. "We're dedicated to meeting every week, weather permitting. We've come from many backgrounds and span a couple generations, but young or old, we have respect for one another both on and off the court. There is a genuine concern about others and what goes on in their daily lives, not just what happens on Thursday nights."

So what happens when there aren't enough players to play a game on Thursday? It is rare, but it does happen. Most likely it happens on those dreary rainy evenings or frosty nights where you'd rather stay in by the fire. There are nights when we will play two-on-two until we cannot move. If less than four players show up, you can rest assured Fran will have some type of basketball-related game to play.

"One time, Fran, Pat Hanlon and I were the only ones there," Mike Brunner recalled. "We played a number of games of free-for-all. Whoever has the ball is on offense against the other two. What a workout! I remember being so tired that I felt like I was going to throw up."

There is also a game called Threes. Often, this game is played as we're waiting for one more player to get a real game started. It's a simple game: the first to make five three-pointers is the winner. It's a tiring game as you can spend much of it chasing long rebounds down the driveway or into the neighbor's yard. What makes it fun is that any ball is a free ball. Take the one closest to you and make the other guy run.

My favorite "alternate" game to play is "Tip HORSE." Fran and I play this a lot, either when we have free time together on Tuesday mornings or when we're the only ones present on a wet Thursday night. You play until the other person has ten points against them. You get a point against you either by having a shot of yours tipped in by the other or by not making a shot that your opponent just made [like in the original game of HORSE]. Fran has owned me in this game because of his unbelievable shooting accuracy. I can hang with him in the games because of the tips and my occasional shooting hot streaks. We have had some epic games together. I remember one time we matched each other on twelve consecutive shots. These games can last forever, if we're both shooting well.

Tip HORSE has given me my favorite shot on the court. It used to be Fran's. Right side corner three-pointer. I rarely miss it now, and it's my go-to shot when we need a three to win a game. But it wasn't always like that. I lost a game of Tip HORSE to Fran once 10–0. And all of his shots were corner threes—one from the right side, one from the left. Back to the right and again from the left. Corner shot after corner shot. He didn't miss. I made a few here and there, mostly from the left side, but he kept shooting them. Over and over. I got frustrated. I tried to hang on, but I couldn't match his accuracy. We must have shot thirty or so threes in that game, fifteen from each corner. Fran smelled blood. He knew I couldn't hit that shot consistently.

Every shot I made only delayed the inevitable. He finally finished off the shutout, but I got so angry at myself that I continued to shoot that shot in other games. At home, the only shot I would take when shooting around was the right corner shot. Over and over. I made it my shot because of that shutout. I owe that to Fran because of a butt-kicking I won't soon forget.

We all have a need for Thursday night hoops, and we all get something different from it. But perhaps the most important thing we get is camaraderie. We don't like missing our regular game for anything and we dare not think of the day we can no longer play. We need this game.

Even the threat of disruptive weather can make us anxious.

We all become meteorologists during the week, constantly updating our weather apps to see the latest forecast. We check down to the hour—Thursday, nine o'clock in the evening. We watch and update radar maps to see if there will be any break in the great green glob heading northeast toward Cincinnati. We do this because bad weather is really the only thing that can stop us from coming.

But even the threat of inclement weather rarely keeps us home.

COME RAIN OR SHINE

> Summer is delicious, rain is refreshing, wind braces up, snow is exhilarating; there is no such thing as bad weather, only different kinds of good weather.
>
> —John Ruskin

Fran sat at his desk in his law office on the west side of Cincinnati. The phone had been ringing all morning. His secretary's voice had been echoing throughout the intercom system, reminding him about meetings, projects, and phone calls still needing to be returned. He had wills to prepare, newsletters to edit, and presentations to write. But nothing could take the hop out of Fran's step. It was, after all, Thursday.

He smiled at the mere thought of it, sitting in his chair and leaning back. But something unnerving caught his eye. He turned toward the window. The cold gray sky had decided to open up and large fluffy flakes had begun to dance toward the ground. The once green grass and dreary gray sidewalks quickly became gleaming white.

He knew what that meant. It was time to make some phone calls.

No, he wasn't going to call the other ball players to let them know that the basketball game would be canceled—how could they play in what was forecasted to be up to an inch or two of snow? That thought, though, never crossed Fran's mind. The snow would end in time. His phone calls were to his daughters whom he knew were home from school.

"Hey, Anne," he said through the receiver to his middle daughter—the one who would one day work full-time as an attorney at his office. "I will need you and Chrissy and Jeanne to shovel the basketball court for me. I won't be home in time to do it before we play tonight. Thanks."

If there was any reluctance on the part of his daughters, Fran didn't know about it. They were used to it by then. They may have been mumbling under their frozen breath as they shoveled load after load of snow off of the court so that it would be dry by nine, but they would not dare tell their dad they wouldn't clear it for Thursday night hoops. They were smarter than that.

"I am pretty amazed at how much attention I have given to Thursday night hoops," Fran said after recalling his earlier days playing this game. "I never think a lot about it, but when I look back and see how much basketball determined how I bought two of my houses and my asking the girls to shovel snow for me, I have to shake my head and laugh to myself."

Snow or no snow, the games would go on.

IT'S NOT THAT BAD OUT THERE

During the winter—before the game eventually moved to a local gymnasium during the frigid months—the players had a rule: If it was twenty degrees or more, the game was on.

"However, some nights would get down to about seventeen degrees and we'd call each other," Fran said. "Let's just play."

So they would show up in sweatshirts and hoods and gloves and snow pants. Shots would refuse to fall because of their puffy gloves. If a shot would go in, they'd have to get a pole or a rake or something similar to poke the ball out of the frozen net. [No one in this group could jump high enough to get it themselves!]

The basketballs would be kept inside the house by a heating vent to keep them from getting flat. If one began to lose bounce during the game, a timeout would be called to switch with one of the balls inside.

The rule may have originally been twenty degrees, but Wayne remembered it was lowered to fifteen degrees. The bottom line: Who cares if it's cold? Get your butt out on the court.

"We'd play in hats and coats, gloves, and layers of clothing," Wayne said. "We'd be numb from the cold but would play on. We played in all kinds of weather. Fran has been known to blow the snow off the court and salt the driveway on Thursdays."

It wasn't always snow that interfered with a perfectly good Thursday night. Sometimes it would rain. And if it rained, any dips or uneven spots on the court would fill with water, creating dead spots on the court. Defenders could set up traps to get the dribbler by one of the puddles in order to force a turnover. In outdoor basketball, you use anything you can to gain an edge.

On rainy evenings, Fran would begin the night by walking the court with huge beach towels to soak up the rain. And between games, everyone would grab a towel and mop up any collected water, each mopping up the area they wanted clean. For me, it's the right corner three-pointer. Puddles tend to fill that area, so I like to spend some extra care and attention there.

"There is no better site than ten grown men with towels bending over and pulling the towels along to dry the court for play," Wayne said. "And on the old court [on Derby], the blacktop portion of the court created a unique experience when it was wet. People would slide all over the court."

Sometimes, playing in the rain was just what the doctor ordered.

"One of my favorite nights started out in typical fashion with six to eight guys showing up," Fred Miller remembered. Fred was one of the original players. "We played several games and some of the guys had to leave. It started to drizzle. The four of us remaining—Fran, Wayne, Greg and I—kept playing, and it kept raining. It was refreshing. The puddles got bigger, but we didn't stop. We just continued on for probably another hour, drenched and having a great time."

The bad weather that many of the guys actually look forward to playing in is the soupy, miserable humidity of early August that resembles steam rooms in local gyms. No matter how hot or humid it gets, it just feels great—especially when the game was played on Derby, the house with the pool.

Back then—before common sense prevailed—the two sides would play shirts vs. skins instead of using red and non-red jerseys. That was a mistake. Some of these guys wore natural sweaters and were soaked in sweat on the drive over. If you've ever seen the movie *Along Came Polly*, you'll understand. The scene where Ben Stiller is playing a game of pick-up basketball outdoors against shirtless behemoths in the blazing sun provides a glimpse of what it can be like. Stiller goes up for a shot. The hairy man leaps for a block and slides his sopping belly down Stiller's face in slow motion. When that happens, it's always in painful slow motion.

"It was pretty gross guarding some of those guys," Wayne remembered.

But they all put up with it because sweet relief was just around the corner.

"I remember stripping off our clothes and jumping in Fran's swimming pool after a long night of hoops," Wayne said. "On particularly hot nights, if we had an odd number, some of us would even jump in the pool to cool off if it was our game to sit out."

Fran needed just one word to describe the relief of the pool.

"Delightful. It was absolutely delightful," he said. "We'd finish playing ball and turn out the lights. Everybody would go on the deck, strip down, and hop in and melt into that pool. It was just delightful on those hot August nights."

Sometimes, however, the cool of the pool isn't the relief needed on a particular Thursday night. Sometimes, relief needs to come on a deeper level.

And sometimes that relief comes just by showing up to simply play a game with some familiar faces.

THERAPY SESSION

> When I step onto the court, I don't have to think about anything. If I have a problem off the court, I find that after I play, my mind is clearer...It is like therapy."
>
> —Michael Jordan

With eyes trained on the road and the traffic around him, Fran was close to completing a lengthy drive from Canada to his home in Cincinnati. His back was tired, but he knew he didn't have a lot to do in the evening other than suit up for basketball. It was Thursday and that was the reason he chose that day to drive home.

He was near the home of a friend who had taken the trip with him when his cell phone rang in the cup holder of his silver Ford Clubwagon. He picked up the phone and said, "Hey, Jim," recognizing the number of his older brother.

"Fran," Jim said, his voice drained and somber at the other end of the line, "Mom died."

After a pause, Jim said more, but Fran didn't hear a word of it. The only words that mattered at that moment were the words he was not ready to hear. Nothing prepares you for the news that a parent has passed away and suddenly, Fran lived in world without his mother.

Mae Niehaus had been sick and in the hospital, but death certainly had not been imminent. The news left Fran numb and looking for answers.

Fran dropped off his friend at his home and then hurried to the hospital to meet his siblings. Tears flowed as stories filled the air-conditioned hospital room where they all gathered. At roughly 9:00 p.m. on that Thursday, Mae's family embraced each other as they said their good-byes for the night. They would see a lot of each other in the coming days. Fran returned to his van, his eyes tired and red, and began the twenty-five-minute drive to Apple Ridge Lane.

"I can't stop thinking about my mom's death," Fran said about his drive home. "But then I realize it's a Thursday, and my thoughts turn to hoops."

Fran continued his drive and pulled onto Apple Ridge Lane. He saw the glow of the lights, which offered some semblance of relief. But then he wondered to himself how or even if he would tell the rest of the players about his mom. He just wanted to play, to do anything he could to take his mind off of the pain.

"We don't really talk a lot about our families out there [on Thursdays]," Fran said. "We just play ball. But despite that, I know there is a lot of care and love."

Fran pulled the van over on the side of the street at the base of his driveway and sauntered slowly up the drive. He nodded hello to a few of the guys and as he somberly approached the garage, "Big" Mike Kraine—who is known for his blunt approach and joking manner—looked over at Fran.

"You're looking a bit glum there, Fran," Mike said, obviously not knowing what Fran had gone through.

Mike's comment made Fran's decision of whether to tell them or not or how to tell the guys a little easier.

"My mom died today, Mike," Fran simply said.

Mike's face twisted into that foot-inserted-squarely-in-mouth look that we've all showcased a time or two in our lives. How could he have known?

"I don't remember much else from that night," Fran said.

I do, though. What happened the rest of the night is one of my fondest and most special memories of my time playing basketball with this group of guys on Thursday nights.

BASKETBALL AS THERAPY

I had known about Fran's mother passing away but felt it should be Fran's news to share. Once he told Mike and everyone knew, I walked over to Fran and gave him a hug. It was hard to see him knowing what he had just gone through. Many of the others stopped shooting around and came over to hug him as well. We may not have known what to say to him—who does?—but he knew that this group was there for him. This group provided Fran the two things that could have eased his pain, even if just a little, that night: basketball and community.

Fran went into the house and emerged a few moments later dressed in his reversible jersey and black shorts and high tops. The feeling of pain was palpable and written all over his body but was there anyone who doubted that Fran would play that night? Certainly no one who has ever shared the court with him.

Fran has always been an incredible shooter. His range has few limits. On that night, however, he had no limitations. Shot after shot swished through the nylon. It didn't matter if he was twisting and turning on reverse layups or stepping out from twenty-five feet, his shots were going down.

Sometimes with tears welling in his red eyes and defenders closing in his face, Fran would drill a shot. Three after three. Shot after shot. Gamer after gamer. It was certainly an inspired effort, one that was absolutely inspiring to me.

It was in that moment, that night, when I realized what a healing impact basketball can have on someone. Basketball is more than a game—it transports you to another world where pain and stress and worries take a seat at the end of the bench. For those three hours that night, Fran could delay the inevitable. Sure the pain would come back, and he would eventually have to lie in bed awake in the dark. Sure the loving memories of his mother would cause pain at the loss and emptiness. But how valuable were those three hours he had to simply shoot a basketball and kick all of our butts that night?

Dr. Mark Smaller, a psychoanalyst who practices in Chicago and Saugatuck, Michigan, certainly understands the therapy that basketball can provide. He uses the game as a form of therapeutic treatment. He explained the need for Fran to play basketball with his friends on the night his mother died, and discussed how basketball and community helped to begin a healthy mourning process.

"I think that in the midst of that kind of traumatic shock—and certainly [his mother's death] would be categorized as a trauma—when you're in that kind of trauma or a semi-traumatic state, you want to be somewhere where you feel most comfortable, where you feel most connected, and where you feel you are most familiar with those around you," Dr. Smaller said. "And it starts a kind of mourning process. Nothing facilitates this mourning process more than being with those you feel most connected to, and connected to in a very particular way."

Dr. Smaller has seen the magic of basketball in action with those who have little else going for them.

Nestled inside Cicero, Illinois, one of the state's oldest municipalities, is Morton Alternative High School, a place of learning near Chicago where students come after expulsion from area high schools for violent and gang-related behaviors. The students attending Morton are fraught with multiple internal and external problems and have not been effectively reached by any other interventions. These students know Morton is their "last stop" and that if they cannot make it at Morton, there is nowhere else for them to go.

Dr. Smaller is on the faculty of the Chicago Institute for Psychoanalysis and the Institute for Clinical Social Work. He is also the founder of Project Realize—formerly the Analytic Service to Adolescents Program [ASAP]—which began as a joint project of Morton Alternative School and the Chicago Institute for Psychoanalysis. According to the Project Realize mission statement, "the central goal of the project is to foster the healthy psychological, social, and educational development of the high-risk student participants, with a specific focus of helping them to achieve graduation from high school."

This program provides in-school psychoanalytic individual and group psychotherapy to students, and ongoing consultation with teachers, staff and parents, and, according to Dr. Smaller, uses the "forward edge" approach.

"The forward edge approach really grows out of a particular psychoanalytic set of theories, but it really focuses on the individual's impulse and instinct to move forward in their lives," he said.

Dr. Smaller provided an example of when he first started at the school nearly ten years ago. A new student arrived at the school, one who was not functioning well and who had a long history of violence related to gangs, and teachers asked the question, "What is wrong with this student?"

"That way of thinking is what we call a trailing edge approach," Dr. Smaller said. "What we try to train our teachers to think about is, it's not what's interfering with this student's functioning, it's what's bringing this student to school. He's coming to school for some reason. If we figure out what that reason is and give him more of that, then we can be successful in helping him in terms of functioning. We reduce the levels of anxiety and depression that can often lead to violent behavior."

One of the ways Dr. Smaller and his program do this is through an after-school basketball program; the pull of the sport, he noticed, can be stronger than the temptation of gang participation

Katie Romey, associate director and psychotherapist at Project Realize, was a social work intern in 2010 and worked with Dr. Smaller at Morton where she facilitated the after-school basketball program. A former basketball player at Cornell, Romey was quite familiar with the therapy basketball could provide and understood the effects of teamwork and cooperation.

"That's what so great about basketball," Dr. Smaller said. "In basketball, when a team is effective, it's not one person, it's the combination of the whole team. Katie is a former basketball player and has coached before. She knows how to facilitate that kind of team approach. A lot of our students at the school have an opportunity to feel part of something at the school, part of a group that actually cares about them."

These students have no shortage of familiarity with group activity; however, the bulk of it deals with gangs and a false sense of belonging.

"One of the things about gangs that is so attractive is that you end up feeling like you are important in the minds of these other guys," Dr. Smaller said. "But the problem with gangs is that you pay a price in terms of having to do illegal or violent things in order to stay a part of that group."

In basketball, however, the feeling of togetherness is nothing but positive. The only negative is that it has to end at some point.

Dr. Smaller's love for basketball gets to mingle with his affection for psychoanalysis every now and then in the form of a student-versus-faculty basketball game at Morton as part of Katie's after-school basketball program. In this game, Dr. Smaller can see firsthand the effects of the game on his students.

Dr. Smaller wrote an article detailing one of these games that occurred in 2010 for *Psychology Today*. In it, he wrote, "Whether playing in a game, or sitting around the gym watching, laughing, or cheering, 'my kids,' as I refer to them, were completely in the moment and having fun. The violence on the street [some students recently lost a friend in a neighborhood shooting], the difficulties at home, and past trauma, were left at the door. Never has so much noise been so soothing to my ears and heart."

Perhaps that is the essence of basketball. It is a joyful gathering of a community forgetting the stresses of the world by working together to accomplish something enjoyable. In his article, Dr. Smaller told the story of a boy who was a player in Katie's program. During the basketball games, he kept receiving phone calls from "his boys," asking where he was. He repeatedly told them he was on his way, but when he would hang up, he continued playing basketball. That court, that game was his safe haven. He wasn't going to leave it for anything.

Basketball–1, Gang life–0.

That sense of community is one of the highlights of the basketball program according to Dr. Smaller. His students represent roughly seven or eight different gangs and, outside of school, they would not even be able to say hello to each other on the street. Through the basketball program and the school environment, these students have developed friendships with each other. Dr. Smaller said he sees basketball as the carrot at the end of the stick that keeps these kids on the right track.

"The power of a group over time, and even over a short time, the cohesiveness that a group can develop and the impact it can have on the individuals in that group is huge," he said. "There is no substitute for it. It's incredibly satisfying and not only in an individual way, it does provide a sense of belonging, a sense of community, and that kind of connection, especially in today's world, is not so easily found. When it is, people get addicted to it. It facilitates a kind of individual growth, and I'm more convinced of that after seeing our kids in the basketball program."

Basketball has provided these troubled youths something special. It is a release for these kids and the joy is obvious and can be felt throughout the gymnasium. But can basketball have the same effect on those who come from solid backgrounds? Those with a solid collection of quality friends and family? Those who already understand and receive the benefits of a positive community?

In a word, absolutely.

Dr. Smaller closed his article by writing, "Basketball has become more than basketball at our school. I can't think of a better way to apply psychoanalytic ideas in the school and out in the world. And that fifty-nine-year old psychoanalyst playing ball? He scored the winning shot and felt sixteen again."

One does not have to have a history of violence or connection to gangs to gain the benefits of basketball. Dr. Smaller felt the positive energy after playing. He felt like a kid again. Everyday stresses from health concerns to financial troubles and from family management to job insecurities can mount just the same. And basketball is there to lend a helping hand. But what is it about the game or about the exercise that allows for this release?

Dr. Smaller certainly has experienced this therapy through playing basketball, but he used an example of another form of activity to help explain the peace that comes through physical activity and working together with others.

There was a fundraising event in Dr. Smaller's home town of Saugatuck, Michigan, called *Dancing for the Arts*. This program raised money for a local arts program and Dr. Smaller was persuaded to take part. He and his dancing partner, a third grade teacher at the local elementary, practiced and rehearsed for six weeks to get ready for the event.

"I had never danced like this," Dr. Smaller said. "It became such a focus for me. Because I was not familiar with this sort of thing, it took my mind, for an hour a week, off of everything else. It turned out to be fun."

After the event, the instructor at the local dance studio where Dr. Smaller's daughters took lessons commented that he had become quite the dancer. She asked the doctor, who privately had held an interest in tap dancing, if he would be interested in participating in a class, if she were to put it together to fit his schedule. Despite never taking a class and not wanting to do any recitals, Dr. Smaller agreed.

Two-and-a-half years later, he is still dancing and has actually participated in two recitals. Dr. Smaller explained why he has continued with the class.

"It is the most relaxing hour of my week when I take that class," he said. "I think it's similar to when I play basketball. When I play basketball, my focus is on my shot, my defense, everything but my normal routine. It's the same with the tap classes; there's nothing else on my mind, and therefore, it becomes the most relaxing time of the week. It is like a moratorium, a timeout."

The same can be said for our group on Thursday nights. Basketball has become more than basketball as Dr. Smaller said. There is a high that is attained, one that becomes almost a necessity.

"The high is not just physical; the high has something to do with feeling, in a very satisfying way, a connection to other people," Dr. Smaller said. "And that is not easy to come by with the demands of everyday life, with work, and family. It really is a kind of timeout, a weekly regrouping of one's thoughts, feelings, and behavior. [This high] provides a kind of mental sustenance before you go back to your normal life."

We may not all have experienced the death of a parent, but we've all come to realize the therapy that is Thursday night hoops at one time or another. The court is a sanctuary. Nothing else matters on the court except for the man guarding you, your teammates on the floor, and that iron basketball hoop awaiting your shot.

This Thursday night group gives each other a rare gift every week—competition and camaraderie. Some of us deal with deadlines and tough clients at work. Some of us work long hours and sacrifice time with family members to support our families financially. Some of us battle sickness and injury. Some of us are worn down by the stresses and exhaustion of raising a young family. Time for ourselves comes fewer and farther between these days. That explains the "need" for this game. Pat Hanlon said that the weekly meeting on the court is one of his fondest memories.

"It's a man-to-man thing," he said. "There's not much that men do together. If they do, it's usually some kind of organization and not something spontaneous. Normally males aren't overly social until they do get together.

"This game, this basketball get-together was an attraction to that male bonding," Pat continued. "We all wanted the same thing. There was an attraction to that male companionship and that strong sense of competition that we all desired. Getting that aggression out or any frustrations out on the court instead of at home was a good thing."

Each of us out there on that court is searching for a sort of refuge from the real world. We are all out there for our own individual reasons—exercise, perspective, fun, therapy, or to simply hit the reset button.

There are two obstacles, however, that can derail that needed peace we seek.

THE INEVITABLES: INJURIES AND DISPUTES

> The body has a stronger memory than the mind.
>
> —Mikhail Baryshnikov

Fran received the ball on the left wing a few feet behind the white, painted-on three-point line. The wind was softly, yet consistently, breathing, but Fran knew that the two-story brick house just behind him would protect his shot from any shenanigans the wind had in store. His defender knew this too and inched even closer, knowing Fran had no fear about shooting from that far away. That night, however, Fran had a different idea.

He dribbled toward the baseline and then weaved in the direction of the basket, wriggling through a crease only he could see or fit into. Drawing a foul he shifted the ball into his right hand and flipped a hook shot high off the backboard as he fell to the ground. The ball skipped off of the backboard and fell through the net. And one!

"Man, how I love a three the old-fashioned way," Fran said. "And this one was a headshaker. The defensive players just shook their head in disbelief when it went in. It was so satisfying."

But playing in the tangled jungle of defenders in the paint increases the odds of landing funny or bouncing the wrong way off of a defender. Too much time in the paint increases the odds of pain—a lesson Fran would learn on his next venture inside where the trees roam.

Feeling inspired by his last shot, Fran had eyes for more inside. He sprinted into the lane to rebound a missed shot from one of his teammates. He lifted for the rebound and landed on a defender's foot, his body wedged between two players. He had nowhere to go but down; the entirety of his weight crushed his ankle. It was unlike any ankle injury he had suffered. He crumpled to the ground like a stadium imploding as the players separated to see what happened.

Unable to walk, Fran literally crawled off of his court, climbed into his house and onto a chair in his kitchen, and sat, immediately wondering how long he would be out. He placed a bag of ice on his already swollen ankle, not fully aware that he was about to face his toughest challenge in the thirty years he had been playing basketball.

THE COMEBACK TRAIL

Fran tore multiple ligaments in his ankle that night in 2013 and underwent more than three months of therapy before he was able to step foot on the court again on Thursday evenings. It was by far the longest he had ever had to sit out on Thursday—the pain of missing almost fourteen weeks of games far outweighed the sting of torn ligaments.

During the Thursday nights that followed the injury, Fran, his lower leg encased in a light-gray walking boot, would come out and mingle with the other players before the games started. He would watch the games for a few minutes before limping inside for the night. It pained him to watch, knowing he couldn't take part. Some nights, he would sit in his living room, a chair propped in front of the window, so he could watch the games.

I knew how he felt. I had been there before.

Four years earlier, I was playing touch football with a lot of the same guys on the brilliant green artificial field turf of St. Xavier High School's practice field. We had played four games, and someone suggested we play another. We all agreed to play one final game. On the first play of the last game, I ran a simple five yard up-and-out route. When I turned the corner, my right foot stayed planted in the field turf as my body spun in the other direction. At first, I thought the quarterback had thrown the football at the back of my ankle. When I turned and saw he still had the ball, I collapsed to the ground.

My Achilles tendon had ruptured; the pop was sickening as was the sight of the tendon curling into my calf.

The worse news that followed the Achilles injury—as with most of our injuries—was the length of time I had to give up basketball. I was off of my feet for a little more than four months, I began shooting again after five months, and it was about half a year before I played on Thursday night again.

Sitting around on Thursday night and then hearing Fran's stories from the games the next day was almost more painful than the injury itself.

Now, with his ankle bulging and discolored, Fran was beginning to see what I had gone through. The game, the community, the involvement in something like this is truly special, and when taken away, the loss can be devastating. We all know how good this Thursday night game is, but we only fully realize its value to us when it is ripped away from us.

Dr. Michael Zito said that Fran's emotion of having to miss out on playing was the result of a strong personal connection to the game and to those with whom he played.

"He benefits a lot from this type of group support, and [with the injury] it's like he has been kicked out of his group therapy," Dr. Zito said. "In that sense, there's a sense of loss. It's important to him because he takes pride in this group; in a sense, it is kind of like his baby. He wants to be involved. He gets a strong sense of enjoyment from playing basketball, which leads to positive emotions and, with the injury, he's not able to get them. With injuries like this, you immediately think, *What if I don't come back.*"

And that is the disturbing thought that accompanies most of our injuries. Mike Brunner, once a regular player whose physical presence was felt with every hard-earned rebound, understands the devastating effect of an injury on the basketball court.

"He was always good to have on your team because of his rebounding and his ability," Fran said. "He was great around the basket."

One night on Fran's court, Mike made a move and awkwardly twisted his knee. He knew almost immediately that he was in trouble.

"That was the most painful thing I have ever felt," he remembered.

He had completely torn his ACL that night, ending his Thursday night playing days with one simple move.

"I'd still be playing if it weren't for the injury," Mike said. "Not being able to play anymore is one of my biggest disappointments. I really loved it. It was one of those regular things I looked forward to every week, a time to just go out and play a game and have fun with a bunch of good people."

John has also had a close call on the court, though he is still able to play on a regular basis. "Big" John is not an ironic nickname. He's big. He's strong. He can effectively box you out with his forearm. When he guards me, I am rendered useless anywhere near the paint.

One of Fran's neighbors decided to play one evening, and this guy took the "big" right out of John's name.

"This guy was a bruiser," John recalled. "He was about six foot four and a lean 260 pounds. He made me look small."

John is a crafty defender. He may not look swift, but he's smart. He'll play to your weakness or try to force you into a predicament. That's how he played the massive neighbor that night.

"I was kind of overplaying him to one side and then snuck around to the other," John said. "So, he thought that side was open, and he just barreled into that side. I had already snuck over there, and I caught his shoulder in the middle of my chest."

John went tumbling back what, he said, felt like five feet. His feet left the ground, and he knew he was headed for a crash landing. He instinctively put his hands down to help break the fall.

"I heard it snap when I hit," John said about his left arm. "It was the most intense pain I had ever felt. I knew it was broken. Like I said, I heard the snap."

Wayne has battled back from a lot to play on Thursday nights. It's remarkable to see how well he still plays, knowing his injury history.

Wayne had lower back surgery in 1998, which he is convinced stemmed from previous jobs and softball games. He missed nine months for that. He had arthroscopic knee surgery to clean his meniscus and missed three months for that. Wayne most recently underwent prostate surgery and missed three or four months.

"I've always said, I'd play until a surgery was repeated on the same body part," Wayne said, who's running out of body parts to cut. "It's hard to miss the games for injury or any reason. For injuries, you know you have to stay away, but you work extra hard to get back to playing as quickly as possible. I visit sometimes when I'm out for a few weeks, just because the guys mean so much. It's in my blood."

Stepping back onto the court after an injury is a different struggle altogether. The doctors may have cleared you physically, but mentally, it's much harder. This was witnessed in the 2012 NBA season when Chicago's Derrick Rose missed the entire year after suffering an ACL tear in the playoffs in the prior season. He was physically cleared to play by team doctors toward the end of the season but refused to play until he was mentally ready. He didn't log a single minute that year, including the postseason.

"It is important where you focus your attention," Dr. Zito said. "A lot of times with injuries, you tend to replay the injury again in your head over and over like a little video tape. Then you play tentatively because you don't want to recreate that injury."

That's what I did when I came back from the Achilles injury. I knew I was physically able to play, but I was far too focused on my right ankle. I had it protected with a high-end brace, but I couldn't erase the sound of the pop from my head. It took a long time before I could drive the lane without thinking about the injury. It certainly affected how I played, even though the tendon had fully recovered.

Dr. Zito, who also plays in a regular basketball game, has dealt with the effects of a serious injury. He tore his ACL and had to overcome that injury in order to continue his playing days.

"I played tentative myself," he said about returning to the court. "But as you continue to go out there, you change your focal point back to the game. That's really what you've got to do. You start out slow, and it's reasonable to start out slow. You have to work to take your focal point off of the injury because that's what makes you tentative, which increases your chances of hurting yourself. It's a matter of refocusing to the task, which is the game of basketball and how it is played."

BOILING POINT

It is a common understanding in basketball that when a team is at game point, they don't get a layup without a foul. It is preferred that they don't even get the shot off if they are anywhere in the paint. As a player on the team at game-point, you expect a foul. You know it's coming. If you drive the lane, you prepare yourself for the contact.

But what happens when a player engages in that foul-at-all-costs battle plan when the score is, say, 10–0 in a game to 20?

"I've only asked one player to leave because of aggressive play," Fran said.

In that case, the score of the game had reached 10-0 and this one particular player was on the team that had yet to score. He, likely, was one of the Game Seven Guys.

He took it upon himself that the leading team would have to earn each and every bucket from that point on. And by earn, he meant survive a barrage of intentional fouls that bordered on assault.

"He went into this hunker-down, beat them up basketball," Fran said. "The next five times the ball went into the lane, he hacked the person trying to get to the hoop and tempers began to...you could just see people getting fired up. You could sense the frustration. It wasn't going to go anywhere good if that continued."

The guys survived the night, but at the end of the games, Fran asked the Ron Artest [or Metta World Peace, is it now?] of the group to take three months off to think about what the game was really about. There was no need to take the game to that level, and clearly, he needed time to cool down. Apparently, three months wasn't enough for him to see the light because that night was the last time he showed up to play.

"I valued the game too much," Fran said. "I liked his friendship, but I valued the game more than to let the game slip into lack of decorum or civility. It was going to be played right."

Only one other person was asked not to attend, but it had nothing to do with aggressive play. It did, however, have to do with injury prevention.

Awhile back, there was a guy who was in need of male bonding and liked the idea of guys getting together every Thursday for basketball and physical activity. There was one problem, however.

"This guy had no athletic talent whatsoever," Fran recalled.

It took only one night for the rest of the players to realize what they were up against. Fran tried to fix the issue by setting up teams so that it was four-on-three with the idea that this new player wasn't going to score at all. The new guy would be all-time defense, similar to how, when we were kids, there was always an all-time snapper when we played football.

"That lasted a very short time because it was clear after that experiment that someone was going to get killed," Fran said. "He just had no idea what the flow of a basketball game looked like. He was always headed in exactly the wrong direction."

The players explained that it just wasn't going to work out and he understood.

"It was unfortunate that he didn't get to get his male bonding by playing basketball with us, but there just wasn't a way in the world that this was going to work, so we just ended it," Fran said.

Even when everyone understands the flow of basketball, disagreements and physical aggression can happen. It's the nature of the game. When you beat on guys over and over for years and years, small annoyances can grow and explode like white heads on a teenager.

Big Mike has been in the middle of a few scuffles. That tends to happen with guys who don't know their own strength.

"When I first started playing with this group, I tended to be relatively aggressive and would generally play very hard to win," Mike admitted. "Sometimes people got pretty mad at me."

Kevin Walsh in particular.

Kevin is a former high school football player and one who was not overly sensitive to physical contact on the basketball court. He could take it. That only adds fuel to Mike's fire, though. When Mike notices that a guy can bang with him inside, Mike tends to bang back just a bit harder. And harder still. I've also been on the receiving end of that situation.

After one too many hits inside, Kevin reached his breaking point. He shoved Mike out of the way and then threw the basketball at him.

"I simply asked him if he felt better after that," Mike said. "He did, so we went on playing."

And that's how most issues are resolved on our court. Play on.

"There are certain nights when you can tell people are a little edgy," John said. "You can sense the tension in the air sometimes—a lot may not be said, but you can tell by the intensity of the defense or how hard someone is boxing out or driving. But that's part of why we do this thing every Thursday night."

Wayne agreed that issues or hard feelings are worked out on the court.

"As with any competition, there have been fights," he said. "Tensions run high on rare occasions and the game gets more physical on those nights. Any fierce competition will have some heated exchanges. We've had no fist fights, but some fouls have been a little hard. Some players took a couple weeks off at times to settle down and not have the hard feelings.

"But in the end, it all gets worked out and we come back the next week for another game."

The irony in this is that, yes, sometimes our emotions and our anger come out on the basketball court. But it is our very presence on that court, our playing basketball together that ultimately helps us handle our emotions and learn how to avoid using our anger in a negative way.

This idea is called "response flexibility" in somatic psychology. Brad Kammer, who is a certified Somatic Experiencing Practitioner and associate professor of psychology at Mendocino College in California, said that playing basketball with a familiar group provides each of the players with a stronger ability to self-regulate. He would know; he, too, plays a little basketball.

"Self-regulation is talking about how our nervous system stays in balance," Kammer explained. "When we have a lot of stress, we tend to lose our ability to self regulate, and we lose response flexibility. When someone says something to us or does something to us, we have an automatic patterned response of getting angry or defensive and that can become a really disruptive behavior if that's the only choice or option we have."

When I was younger, my response mechanism was as rigid as a steel goal post. But now, as I've matured and have ten years of experience playing with these guys, I know there are more [better] options than coming at someone defensively, if I feel I've been fouled too hard or if someone says something to me that I take personally. I attribute that growth to a decade of basketball therapy. Perspective has been gained, lessons have been learned. I feel like I have much better control over my emotions than I did when I first started playing with this group.

According to Kammer, playing basketball can provide a release of stress energy. In somatic experiencing, the focus is on the body's ability to self-regulate. The goal is to have an awareness that there is more than one option available to us when responding to someone. It is a biological process, according to Kammer, that's working within each of us, one that filters up through the brain and comes out through words and actions. Kammer said that many different practices from meditative practice to creative or artistic practices to athletics can enhance our ability to self-regulate.

"There is something about basketball that allows all those parts of ourselves that can get fragmented in the daily life to come together," Kammer said. "We talk about in neuroscience, a term called coherence, which refers to when different systems are working together with one another. For me, when you can get into that place in basketball, when all parts of you are working in coordination with one another, everything can work in balance again."

Maybe that is what is commonly referred to as "the zone" in basketball, that feeling of Zen when everything seems to be working perfectly. When that "zone" is disrupted by injury or conflict, it can take a while to get it back.

It's always nice to know there will be a next week to erase the frustrations of injury or the remorse after a disagreement. But, in the distance, there lives that unpleasant thought of a Thursday night that won't include basketball, that first Thursday that comes around after you take your high-tops off for the final time.

CLOSING TIME

> For when the One Great Scorer comes to write against your name, He marks—not that you won or lost—but how you played the game.
>
> —Grantland Rice

It was 11:52 p.m., and the six remaining players struggled to stand upright. Our jerseys were soaked, our water bottles were empty, our ankles and knees were screaming. Each team had won a game in the final series of the night.

"Championship of the world," Wayne said, standing at the top of the key awaiting the check for the final game of the night. No one wanted to end the night with a loss.

The game progressed as did the first two with each team fighting for points. Jumpers were just short, layups were missing the mark, passes were not finding their intended targets. But we trudged on. Each team was scrapping for inside points, usually coming on put-backs after missed shots. One team neared the finish line, pushing closer to the end on the strength of a few three-pointers that managed to find the inside of the hoop.

We could tell the game's end was near because Fran, on the trailing team, began to do the calculations in his head.

"Okay, we need two threes and two twos," he yelled to his teammates as he dribbled with the ball. "In any order!"

Whenever his opponent is one or two scores from the finish line, Fran is known to lay out the game plan.

"He is always calculating what we need to pull out the win," Wayne said. "We always know how many threes we need."

Even with exhaustion taking over our bodies, the last game of the rugged night ended with a flourish, a grand finale.

All of a sudden, the game was tied at eighteen after the trailing team, running on fumes, took advantage of the defense's sluggish feet and nailed a few open shots. The next team to score would be the winner. We all knew this was Wayne's time of night, but somehow, he still managed to find a hole just outside of the paint. Jason rifled him the ball and Wayne's shot was as smooth as silk. Game over.

Night over. Sweet relief.

WHEN THE LIGHTS GO OUT

There are few greater moments during the week than when a game hangs in the balance—next shot wins—on a Thursday night.

And when you are the one who is fortunate enough to sink a gamer, that little positive buzz tends to stay with you for a while. We've each had one; the most satisfying game-enders are the ones that finish exhausting games late in the evening.

When the games are over for the night, some of us will lie flat on our backs, staring at those white spots, hovering above like glowing gnats. Some of us will go through our stretching routine so that we'll be able to walk in the morning. There is usually some chatter about the night filled with compliments and hopefulness at the idea that shots may fall a little more frequently the next week.

And then it's clean-up time. The flood lights on the pole must come down—a much more difficult task at the end of the night. Basketballs are put away, chairs back in their place. A roll call of who will be or won't be here the next week takes place and we'll all say our good-byes after another beautiful night.

I'm always thankful at that moment for survival. I sit in my minivan, enjoying that beautiful peace that comes only when sitting for the first time in three hours. I take a few deep breaths and relax as the other cars, one by one, turn around and head back up the hill of Apple Ridge Lane, their headlights fading to black. I stare out of the windshield and send a little prayer of thanks for getting through the night injury free and for allowing me the chance to play in this game. As mentioned earlier, there is a certain clarity of mind after a great night of basketball. Perspective is more in line. Priorities are in place. All is right with the world. It is right, at that time, to offer up thanks to God for these opportunities—opportunities that not everyone is fortunate enough to have.

And, as I've also mentioned before, there will be that day when the lights turn out on our last night of Thursday night hoops. There will come a Thursday night when we will stay at home for good. There will be a Thursday night when Fran's court of dreams will sit vacant and dark. And accompanying that night will be an emptiness that Pat Hanlon and Mike Brunner and others unfortunately already know all too well.

Greg knows his end could be near but refuses to simply quit on the game he has been an integral part of for thirty years.

"I'll be honest, the last five years, I've been gradually playing less," he said. "When you can't play the way you used to, it can be hard to take. I can't play like I used to because of my knees and my back, and it's a little depressing. But when I take a few weeks off and come back, it's not as big a problem. I'm more rested and can play better. So that's how I'm going to keep playing. I'll just play less. I never thought I'd be playing [this long] anyway."

Fran is in his sixties, but showing no signs of slowing down. He doesn't even want to think about the day he can't play on Thursday nights anymore. I think he would be satisfied walking away from the game the night after playing on Thursday night with his grandson, Aidan, for the first time. I think that is a goal for him—to be competitive enough to play against his grandson.

Aidan is five years old now.

"I feel a lot older today, but I'm only sixty-three, and I keep myself in good shape," Fran said. "I had once thought I'd play until seventy, but I'd like to make it until seventy-three when I could play with Aidan. There was never a doubt that I could play until seventy-five until now [after the ankle injury].

"My ankle scares me, but ankles heal," Fran continued. "Hurting my knee really scares me, but what can I do? I have to keep in shape, pray, and be grateful for every Thursday night I have."

Roger's goal was to play until he turned fifty.

"That was [seven] years ago," Roger said. "Then, it was age sixty, but that is obviously too soon. So now my goal is to keep playing quality ball as long as Fran and Wayne do."

Roger may have to delay any retirement parties for quite some time, then.

Jason doesn't have a longevity goal but said that seventy would be a nice number, if his knees and back hold out.

Me, I want to play until I have a grandchild that is old enough to play. I want to infuriate him with the same "old guy" tricks that the guys use against me. I am thirty-four now, but Byron Heizer assures me I'm knocking on the door of old-guy status.

Wayne has already said that he'll play until he has surgery on the same body part for a second time. But what if that never happens?

"My goal was and still is, I guess, to play at sixty," Wayne once said.

Wayne turned sixty in September of 2013. He's still playing as well as ever.

"I'm not one to play halfway, so someday, I may have a heart attack on the court," he said. "I always said if that happens, just roll me off the court and play on."

The game has waned a bit recently; Father Time can be quite a lockdown defender. As some players age, muscles and joints nag just a little louder and a little more frequently. Weariness becomes more noticeable. And if old age doesn't get the best of some, life changes can also keep us from the game.

Mike Kraine has moved to Boston; his playing days also cut short by painful knees. Byron White is struggling with Achilles injuries and distant travel due to a career in Cleveland. There are some nights, though, when Byron makes that drive from Cleveland on Thursday nights and pulls into Apple Ridge just after nine. He too needs that fix every once in a while. Scott is no longer a regular, every once in a while showing up to capture a little slice of his past. But even though many have called it a career, there is a sense that the game will somehow find a way to continue.

"In our aging, we've moved indoors for our winter play," Wayne said. "We've been to high school gyms, grade school gyms, and public sports centers. Wherever we go the game goes with us. Aside from adding full court running for part of the year now, the game remains the same. Shoot foul shots to determine teams, play best of three, shoot for new teams.

"Players move on, new ones come in, but the game," Wayne said, "will go on."

I, for one, will do my part to make sure he is right. Because, quite frankly, I'm not sure how I could possibly be at my best without the benefits I receive every Thursday night when the clock strikes nine.

The thought of one day not being able to play the game we love scares some of us. But why? Is it the sport itself that we'll miss? Is it the attachment to doing something we all did as kids? Is it those we play against? The community? The highs?

It is all of those.

Psychologist Brad Kammer said that this basketball group is a perfect storm of positive interaction, which makes it almost like an addiction of sorts. It is, and will be, very hard to stop for each of us.

"The first time, if I look back, that I really remember feeling safety in community, was when I played basketball," Kammer recalled. "I think that is a really deep thing.

I didn't have to do anything to be accepted. I just had to show up. They were my tribe.

"All animals, including humans, have an implicit need of having a sense of community," Kammer continued. "Down to fish, they have schools that swim together. There is swarming behavior and herd behavior in animals. Community is something all animals need for survival. Part of the challenge in our society these days is that we don't have that connection to others anymore."

In 2005, following the devastating destruction of Hurricane Katrina, Kammer traveled to New Orleans with a team of specialists to do Somatic work on those struggling with the horrific aftermath. It is in this post-storm chaos where Kammer said he saw just how powerful community can be for those suffering from trauma.

In the immediate aftermath of the historical storm, more than twenty thousand of those displaced from their homes were sent to the Superdome, a massive structure where the New Orleans Saints played their home football games. Instead of passionate screaming fans cheering, the dome was filled with homeless, injured, and the dying. Report after report on national news outlets and 24/7 cable news channels told stories of mayhem, rape, attacks, and horrid sanitary problems that made viewers squeamish.

While in New Orleans, Kammer came across a woman who was on the clean-up crew of the Superdome. While most of the news coverage centered on the horrific acts going on inside the dome, one thing caught the eye of this woman when she was cleaning the mess left inside the dome.

Placed inside the dome on the football field, there were thousands of chairs and cots for those with nowhere else to live. But they weren't in rows like at a recital or sitting haphazardly on the field turf. What she found were several large circles of chairs all over the field. Circle after circle speckled the green field, an image that told the story of how strangers had come together in this traumatic experience to form their own small communities within the Superdome.

"There were a lot of people coming together in community to help deal with the trauma they were going through," Kammer said. "The media completely missed that, of course. Our natural tendency is to come together with people to regulate through our traumas and our grief."

And this group of basketball players comes together every Thursday to help us regulate through our daily stresses, our own personal grief, and our pent up frustrations. Basketball—the sport—isn't the only thing keeping this group together. The bond of community present in basketball plays a great role in the longevity of this Thursday night tradition.

Finding a group like this collection of individuals who have come together now for thirty years to do something they love can be a lifesaver. The release of body chemicals that create a high during exercise coupled with the sense of community can be a powerful thing. And when that's gone, the body and the mind know it.

We have stressful lives and even positive stress can be detrimental to the body and the mind.

"We're dealing with a lot of stuff every day," Kammer said. "It gets us into survival mode and even if the stress is good stress, we all need ways to discharge that survival energy. That's what happens with chronic stress. That energy gets trapped in our bodies and it turns to illness."

Without an opportunity to release that stress, perspective can be lost, among other problems.

"I think, the way that the brain is organized, our perception tends to be based on internal experience," Kammer said. "When the internal experience is given room to shift, then our perception also shifts. And I think, that when you have something that works to help regulate through that energy, it shifts not only your physiological state, but your perceptive state and your intellectual state."

Kammer said that the strong sense of loss when one has to quit playing basketball with the group comes from the inherent needs being met each and every Thursday night. In effect, this group is a microcosm of a happy life.

"We're disconnected in our society, not only in our bodies and minds and our health and stress, but also in the sense that we are disconnected from other people who are supposed to be there to help regulate us," he said. "When you get into an environment such as this basketball group where you're actually working together as a team and you're having fun, I think that really has a deeper level of healing, one you can really only find in a community."

And when that deeper level of healing ceases to exist and that community is no longer a part of your routine, the sense of loss is real. Pat Hanlon knows this all too well.

"[Thursday night hoops] was akin to going to church on Sundays," Pat remembered, looking the way a man does when he wishes he still could do what he loved. He is in his eighties now, a snow-white beard framing his face. Pat played until two knee injuries and multiple surgeries ended his playing career at age sixty-six.

Pat, who also played basketball for the senior Olympic team, said hanging up the high-tops was one of the hardest decisions he's had to make in his life because of what he would be missing, because of what he would never be a part of again.

"The most difficult thing I had to do in my life—other than my divorce—was to give up playing basketball," he said. "[It was] without a doubt, the biggest emotional adjustment I've had to go through. I just got so much out of it. Great support and nurturing. That's another reason guys like to play: You get a real sense of accomplishment. Success. You were accepted. They genuinely wanted you to be there."

And every now and then on a Thursday evening, Pat will finish his supper and clear the table. Settling in for the night, he will pick up a book or will sit down at his computer to do some writing of his own. Deep in thought, he will glance at the clock on the wall and sigh. It will be closing in on nine and Pat will get that itch once again.

"Oh yeah, I still think about it," he said quietly. "On Thursday nights, I still think about the guys out there playing. Thursday night, to me, will always be basketball night. That's just the way it is."

BIBLIOGRAPHY

Bernstein, Lenny. 2010. "MisFits: 20 Years of Pickup Basketball and Still Bonding." *The Washington Post*. Accessed October 14, 2013. http://www.washingtonpost.com/wp-dyn/content/article/2010/12/21/AR2010122102269.html

Dweck, Carol S. Mindset: the new psychology of success. New York: Random House, 2006

Hruby, Patrick. 2007. "The Ultimate Hoops Game from Hell." *Hruby: We Got Next*. Accessed October 13, 2013. http://sports.espn.go.com/espn/page2/story?page=hruby/070517

Hruby, Patrick. 2009. "Hellish Pickup Players, 2.0." *Hruby: We Got Next*. Accessed October 14, 2013. http://sports.espn.go.com/espn/page2/story?page=hruby/070517

"James Naismith Handwritten Manuscript Detailing First Basketball Game." *HA.com*. Heritage Auctions, n.d. Web. Accessed October 14, 2013. http://sports.ha.com/c/item.zx?saleNo=706

Klosterman, Chuck. 2009. "Craig Robinson: America's First Coach." *Esquire.com Article*. Accessed May 2013.

http://www.esquire.com/features/chuck-klostermans-america/obama-basketball-story-0209

Krakovsky, Marina. 2007. "The Effort Effect." *Stanford Magazine*. Stanford University. Accessed October 14, 2013. http://alumni.stanford.edu/get/page/magazine/article/?article_id=32124

McCuaig, Donald S. "Basketball : A YMCA Invention." *YMCA.int*. Accessed October 14, 2013. http://www.ymca.int/who-we-are/history/basketball-a-ymca-invention/

Neel, Eric. "Living and Dying for the Game." *ESPN.com*. Accessed October 14, 2013. http://sports.espn.go.com/espn/eticket/story?page=saturdaygame

"Newly Found Documents Shed Light on Basketball's birth." *ESPN.com*. The Associated Press, 13 Nov. 2006. Accessed October 14, 2013. http://sports.espn.go.com/nba/news/story?id=2660882

Smaller, Mark D., Ph.D. 2010 "Sometimes Basketball Is More Than Basketball: Psychoanalysis Scores a Slam Dunk!" Web log post. *The Analyst in the Classroom*. Psychology Today. Accessed August 23, 2013. http://www.psychologytoday.com/blog/the-analyst-in-the-classroom/201012/sometimes-basketball-is-more-basketball-psychoanalysis-scor